Quality Assurance for Pharmacy-Prepared Sterile Products Workbook

A Multi-Media Self-Instructional Program

Contributing Editors

Toby Clark

Timothy Fox

Greg Snyder

Toby Clark, M.S., is the Director of Hospital Pharmacy Services, University of Illinois at Chicago Medical Center, Chicago, Illinois.

Timothy Fox, Pharm.D., is a Clinical Pharmacist, Jefferson Home Infusion Services, Philadelphia, Pennsylvania.

Greg Snyder, B.S., is the Assistant Director of Pharmacy, Lehigh Valley Hospital, Allentown, Pennsylvania.

Shelley Morse Bethmann provided instructional design consultation.

Produced by the American Society of Health-System Pharmacists' Special Projects Division.

ISBN: 1-879907-46-1

Dear Purchaser:

To purchase and complete the CE program for this product, go to the ASHP CE Testing Center at http://www.ashp.org/ce/. Log in using your Customer ID Number from the purchase invoice or your ASHP Member ID Number. Once you have successfully logged in, follow the instructions provided for completing and submitting your test.

TABLE OF CONTENTS

Introduction 1

Glossary 3

Section One: Aseptic Preparation of Parenteral Products 7
    Overview 7
    Objectives 7
    Discussion Points
        1.1 Laminar air flow 8
        1.2 Syringes and needles 10
        1.3 Vials and ampules 11
        1.4 Preparing IV admixtures 13
    Summary 13
    Tips 14
    Exercises 14
    Self-Assessment Questions 15

Section Two: Introduction to Risk Level Classification 17
    Overview 17
    Objectives 17
    ASHP TAB (Abridged) 18
    Discussion Points 19
    Summary 22
    Exercises 22
    Self-Assessment Questions 23

Section Three: Quality Assurance for Risk Level One 25
    Overview 25
    Objectives 25
    3.1 ASHP TAB (Abridged) 26
    Discussion Points
        3.1 Policies, procedures, and personnel training
            programs 27
    3.2 ASHP TAB (Abridged) 28
    Discussion Points
        3.2 Storage and handling, facilities and
            equipment, garb 30

Exercises 32

Self-Assessment Questions 33

3.3–3.4 ASHP TAB (Abridged) 34

Discussion Points

    3.3 Aseptic technique and product preparation 36

    3.4 Process validation 36

Tips 37

Exercises 37

Self-Assessment Questions 38

3.5 ASHP TAB (Abridged) 39

Discussion Points

    3.5 Expiration dating, labeling, end-product
        evaluation, documentation 40

Summary 42

Tips 42

Exercises 43

Self-Assessment Questions 43

Section Four: Quality Assurance for Risk Level Two 45

Overview 45

Objectives 45

4.1–4.2 ASHP TAB (Abridged) 46

Discussion Points

    4.1 Policies and procedures, personnel education,
        training and evaluation 48

    4.2 Storage and handling, facilities and equipment,
        garb 49

Tips 51

Exercises 51

Self-Assessment Questions 51

4.3–4.4 ASHP TAB (Abridged) 52

Discussion Points

    4.3 Aseptic technique and product preparation 53

    4.4 Process validation 56

Tips 56

Exercises 57

Self-Assessment Questions 57

4.5 ASHP TAB (Abridged) 58

Discussion Points

    4.5 Expiration dating, labeling, end-product
        evaluation, documentation 59

Summary 61

Tips 61

Exercises 61

Self-Assessment Questions 62

Section Five: Quality Assurance for Risk Level Three 63

Overview 63

Objectives 63

5.1 ASHP TAB (Abridged) 64

Discussion Points

    5.1 Policies and procedures, personnel education,
        training and evaluation 65

Tips 67

Exercises 68

Self-Assessment Questions 68

5.2 ASHP TAB (Abridged) 69

Discussion Points

    5.2 Storage and handling, facilities and equipment,
        garb 71

Tips 73

Exercises 73

Self-Assessment Questions 74

5.3 ASHP TAB (Abridged) 74

Discussion Points

    5.3 Aseptic technique and product preparation,
        process validation, expiration dating, labeling,
        end-product evaluation, documentation 76

Summary 80

Tips 80

Exercises 80

Self-Assessment Questions 81

Appendix 1 83
ASHP technical assistance bulletin on quality assurance for
pharmacy-prepared sterile products 85

INTRODUCTION

As pharmacists and pharmacy technicians, you are responsible for the aseptic preparation of sterile products. In order to help you meet and maintain standards that ensure your pharmacy-prepared sterile products are of the highest quality, the American Society of Hospital Pharmacists (ASHP) has designed this interactive program entitled "Quality Assurance for Pharmacy-Prepared Sterile Products."

ASHP has developed recommendations outlined in the "ASHP Technical Assistance Bulletin on Quality Assurance for Pharmacy-Prepared Sterile Products" (Appendix I). The objectives of these recommendations are to provide:

♦ information to pharmacists on quality assurance and quality control activities that may be applied to the preparation of sterile products in pharmacies and;

♦ a scheme to match quality assurance and quality control activities with the potential risks posed to patients.

The program you are about to begin is designed to discuss, in depth, these recommendations, the three levels of risk associated with preparation of sterile products, and how to initiate quality assurance policies and procedures within your own work environment. The information will be presented in an interactive format using a videotape and workbook. The program is divided into five sections:

Section One: Aseptic Preparation of Parenteral Products
Section Two: Introduction to Risk Level Classification
Section Three: Quality Assurance for Risk Level One
Section Four: Quality Assurance for Risk Level Two
Section Five: Quality Assurance for Risk Level Three

You will cover the topic areas at your own pace—in a group setting or on your own. While viewing the videotape, you will be asked to refer to the workbook. You will first read an abridged version of the ASHP Technical Assistance Bulletin (TAB), followed by discussion points. A series of practical exercises and tips are offered to help you apply the information that has been presented. You are then asked to complete self-assessment questions.

How to Use This Program

This program has been designed so that you can work at your own pace. You do not have to complete the exercises while viewing the videotape, but rather familiarize yourself with the content, then return, at a later time, to complete each exercise. Where relevant, you are given a list of supplies you will need to complete the exercises. It is important to complete as many of these exercises as you can in order to apply the principles and information that you have been given in both the text and the manual. The workbook also contains a glossary of terms that you should become familiar with.

You will also notice that icons have been used in sections 3, 4, and 5 of the videotape. These icons are to help you easily recognize which topic and risk level you were at when you paused the videotape.

You should work through this entire program first before reviewing any sections out of sequence. The self assessment questions within each section are written to test your mastery of the subject. Please complete each one and record your answers in this workbook. For continuing education credits, please forward the enclosed CE test answer sheet to ASHP.

You are now invited to begin. Good luck and enjoy the program!

GLOSSARY

Aseptic preparation:
The technique involving procedures designed to preclude contamination (of drugs, packaging, equipment, or supplies) by microorganisms during processing.

Batch preparation:
Compounding of multiple sterile-product units, in a single discrete process, by the same individual(s), carried out during one limited time period.

Cleanroom:
A room in which the concentration of airborne particles is controlled and there are one or more clean zones. (A clean zone is a defined space in which the concentration of airborne particles is controlled to meet a specified airborne-particulate cleanliness class.) Cleanrooms are classified based on the maximum number of allowable particles 0.5 mm and larger per cubic foot of air. For example, the air particle count in a Class 100 cleanroom may not exceed a total of 100 particles of 0.5 mm and larger per cubic foot of air.

Closed-system transfer:
The movement of sterile products from one container to another in which the container-closure system and transfer devices remain intact throughout the entire transfer process, compromised only by the penetration of a sterile, pyrogen-free needle or cannula through a designated stopper or port to effect transfer, withdrawal, or delivery. Withdrawal of a sterile solution from an ampule in a Class 100 environment would generally be considered acceptable; however, the use of a rubber-stoppered vial, when available, would be preferable.

Compounding:
For purposes of this program, compounding simply means the mixing of substances to prepare a medication for patient use. This activity would include dilution, admixture, repackaging, reconstitution, and other manipulations of sterile products.

Controlled area:
For purposes of this program, a controlled area is the area designated for preparing sterile products.

Critical areas:
Any area in the controlled area where products or containers are exposed to the environment.

Critical site:
An opening providing a direct pathway between a sterile product and the environment or any surface coming in contact with the product or environment.

Critical surface:
Any surface that comes into contact with previously sterilized products or containers.

Expiration date:
The date (and time, when applicable) beyond which a product should not be used (i.e., the product should be discarded beyond this date and time). NOTE: Circumstances may occur in which the expiration date and time arrive while an infusion is in progress. When this occurs, judgment should be applied in determining whether it is appropriate to discontinue that infusion and replace the product. Organizational policies on this should be clear.

HEPA filter:
A high-efficiency particulate air (HEPA) filter composed of pleats of filter medium separated by rigid sheets of corrugated paper or aluminum foil that direct the flow of air forced through the filter in a uniform parallel flow. HEPA filters remove 99.97% of all air particles 0.3 mm or larger. When HEPA filters are used as a component of a horizontal- or vertical-laminar-airflow hood, an environment can be created consistent with standards for a Class 100 cleanroom.

Quality assurance:
For purposes of this program, quality assurance is the set of activities used to ensure that the processes used in the preparation of sterile drug products lead to products that meet predetermined standards of quality.

Quality control:

For purposes of this program, quality control is the set of testing activities used to determine that the ingredients, components (e.g., containers), and final sterile products prepared meet predetermined requirements with respect to identity, purity, nonpyrogenicity, and sterility.

Repackaging:

The subdivision or transfer from a container or device to a different container or device, such as a syringe or ophthalmic container.

Sterilizing filter:

A filter that, when challenged with a solution containing the microorganism *Pseudomonas diminuta*, at a minimum concentration of 10^{12} organisms per square centimeter of filter surface, will produce a sterile effluent.

Temperatures (USP):

Frozen means temperatures between –20 and –10 °C (–4 and 14 °F). Refrigerated means temperatures between 2 and 8 °C (36 and 46 °F). Room temperature means temperatures between 15 and 30 °C (59 and 86 °F).

Validation:

Documented evidence providing a high degree of assurance that a specific process will consistently produce a product meeting its predetermined specifications and quality attributes.

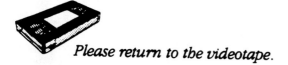

Please return to the videotape.

SECTION ONE: ASEPTIC PREPARATION OF PARENTERAL PRODUCTS

OVERVIEW

In order to ensure the safety of your patients and to use sterile equipment and supplies, you must have an understanding of laminar air flow principles, the proper use of the laminar air flow hood, and development and maintenance of manipulative techniques to prepare sterile parenteral products.

OBJECTIVES

Upon completion of this section, you should be able to:

- Define a "Class 100" environment.

- Explain the 10 principles of the laminar flow hood operation.

- Demonstrate the proper positioning of sterile objects in laminar air flow hood.

- Understand that there are two kinds of laminar flow hoods and how each is used.

- Describe the parts of a syringe and, to maintain sterility, proper handling of a syringe.

- Describe the parts of a needle and how to define needle size.

- Demonstrate the proper technique for handling and attaching sterile needles to syringes.

- Demonstrate the proper technique for opening and removing drug fluid from an ampule.

- Demonstrate the proper procedure for reconstituting a powdered drug in a vial.

- Demonstrate the proper procedure for removing fluid from a vial.

- Demonstrate the proper technique for preparing admixtures in polyvinyl chloride (PVC) bags, glass containers, and semirigid plastic containers.

DISCUSSION POINTS

1.1 Laminar Air Flow

Sterile products should be prepared in a "Class 100" environment, containing no more than 100 particles per cubic foot that are 0.5 micron or larger in size. This "Class 100" environment is achieved with a laminar flow hood with either a horizontal or vertical flow.

The underlying principle of the laminar flow hood is that the constant flow of twice-filtered, laminar sheets or layers of "aseptic" air, at a rate of approximately 90 linear feet per minute across the work surface, physically sweeps the work area and prevents the entry of contaminated room air.

The horizontal flow hood first draws contaminated room air through a prefilter similar to a furnace filter which removes only gross contaminants. The prefiltered air is then pressurized within a plenum to assure that a consistent distribution of air flow is presented to the "HEPA" filter. This "high efficiency particulate air filter" removes 99.9% of particles that are 0.3 micron or larger, thereby eliminating airborne microorganisms.

In vertical flow hoods, HEPA filtered air emerges from the top and passes downward through the work area. Because exposure to some antineoplastic drugs may be harmful, they are usually prepared in biological safety cabinets, which utilize vertical air flow, to maintain sterility and protect the operator.

The critical principle to remember when using a laminar flow hood is that *nothing must interrupt the flow of air between the HEPA filter and a sterile object.* To maintain sterility, nothing should pass behind a sterile object in a horizontal flow hood or above one in a vertical flow hood.

Ten General Principles for Proper Laminar Flow Hood Operation

1. All aseptic manipulations should be performed at least six inches within the hood to prevent the possibility of reflected contamination.

2. A laminar flow hood should be left operating continuously.

3. Before use, all interior working surfaces of the laminar flow hood should be cleaned from back to front, top to bottom, away from the HEPA filter with an appropriate agent (e.g., 70% isopropyl alcohol and clean wipes).

4. Nothing should be permitted to come in contact with the HEPA filter including cleaning solution, aspirate from syringes, or glass from ampules.

5. A laminar flow hood should be positioned away from excess traffic, doors, air vents, or anything that could produce air currents capable of introducing contaminants into the hood.

6. Eating, drinking and smoking is always prohibited. In addition, jewelry should not be worn on hands or wrists when working in the laminar flow hood.

7. Talking or coughing should be directed away from the laminar flow hood working area to minimize air flow turbulence.

8. Only those objects essential to product preparation should be placed in the laminar flow hood.

9. Laminar flow hoods should be tested by qualified personnel every six months, whenever the hood is moved, or if filter damage is suspected.

10. The use of the laminar flow hood alone, without the observance of aseptic technique, cannot insure product sterility.

Please return to the videotape.

1.2 Syringes and Needles

Another important factor in aseptic preparation is the correct use of syringes and needles.

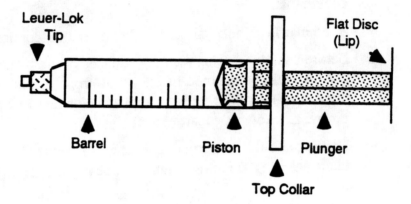

When measuring with a syringe, the final edge (closest to the tip of the syringe) of the plunger piston, which comes in contact with the syringe barrel, should be lined up to the graduation mark on the barrel. To maintain sterility, the syringe tip and plunger should not be touched.

KEY POINTS TO REMEMBER ABOUT SYRINGES

■ syringes are commonly available in sizes ranging from 0.5 to 60 milliliters.

■ graduation marks on syringes represent different increments, depending on size of syringe.

■ to ensure accuracy, do not use a syringe whose graduations are greater than twice the volume being measured.

■ to maintain sterility, neither the syringe tip or the plunger should not be touched.

A needle shaft is usually metal and is lubricated with a sterile silicone coating, so, for this reason do not swab a needle with alcohol.

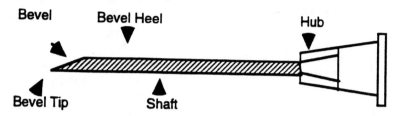

Bevel **Bevel Heel** **Hub**

Bevel Tip **Shaft**

KEY POINTS TO REMEMBER ABOUT NEEDLES

■ needle size is designated by two numbers, measuring gauge and length.

■ the gauge of the needle corresponds to the diameter of the needle's bore and ranges from 27 (finest) to 13 (largest).

■ manipulate needles by their protective covers only. Never touch any part of the needle proper.

■ in order to maintain sterility, open needle package within the laminar flow hood.

The protective covers should be left on both syringes and needles until ready for use. Both syringes and needles are sent from the manufacturer assembled and individually packaged. The sterility of the contents is guaranteed as long as the outer package remains intact. However, packages should always be inspected before using and discarded (in approved safety containers) if damaged.

Please return to the videotape.

1.3 Vials and Ampules

Injectable medications are usually supplied in vials or ampules, each requiring different techniques for withdrawal of the medication.

It is very important to follow these procedures when handling both vials and ampules.

Aseptic Technique for Vials

To prevent contamination	Swab rubber closure with 70% alcohol using firm strokes in same direction.
To prevent core formation	Insert needle to penetrate the rubber closure at same point with both tip and heel of bevel.
To prevent vacuum formation	Because vials are closed-system containers, replace with air the volume of fluid to be removed by injecting a quantity of air equal to the fluid volume.
Reconstituting drug powder	As diluent is added to powder, an equal volume of air must be removed to prevent positive pressure from developing inside vial.

Aseptic Technique for Ampules

To break an ampule properly	Clean ampule neck with alcohol swab, leave swab in place, grasp ampule by neck with thumb and index finger. Use quick, firm, snapping motion away from body. *Do not break toward HEPA filter.*
To withdraw medication from ampule	Tilt ampule, place needle bevel in corner space near opening, pull back syringe plunger to withdraw solution.
To avoid contamination of ampule solution	Use needle with 5-micron filter or filter straw either as solution is pulled into or pushed out of syringe.

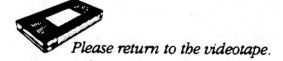

Please return to the videotape.

1.4 Preparing IV Admixtures

It is crucial that good aseptic technique is followed when preparing IV admixtures.

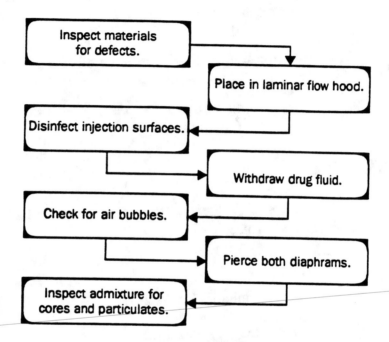

SUMMARY

Aseptic technique is a way of manipulating sterile products without contamination. Hand washing, proper use of the laminar flow hood, and strict aseptic technique are very important factors in preventing the contamination of sterile products. Other important factors include proper syringe handling, the withdrawal of medicines from a vial or ampule, and the filling of IV bags or glass bottles.

TIPS

➤ When handwashing, be sure to remove all rings from your fingers.

➤ When cleaning a hood, be sure to use a small amount of alcohol (70%) or other approved product. Too much is wasteful and may damage the HEPA filter.

➤ When working in a hood, assemble all supplies and components on a 4" x 6" tray before you start the compounding process.

➤ When inspecting a bag for defects, squeeze the bag hard to check for pin holes or leaks.

EXERCISES

In order to complete these exercises, you should have the following materials availaable:

* syringes
* needles
* 10 ampules (1ml and 10ml sizes)
* filter needles
* 5 vials of lyophilized injection
* PVC bags or glass IV bottles

You should now practice the following functions at least 5 times or until you feel you are competent to demonstrate your proficiency to another person.

1. Opening a syringe from paper overwrap.

2. Opening a needle and placing it on the syringe.

3. Opening an ampule—1 ml and 10 ml. (Be sure you do this 5 times without cutting your fingers.)

4. Using a filter needle to withdraw the contents of the ampules you opened previously. Dispose of the drug in the prescribed manner.

5. Reconstitute a minimum of 5 vials of a lypholized injection. Make sure you do not core the stopper or cause a vacuum or pressure to build up in the completed product.

6. Properly add drug from a vial and ampule to a PVC bag or glass IV bottle.

SELF-ASSESSMENT QUESTIONS

1. Labels can be placed in a laminar flow hood.
   a. True
   b. False

2. A laminar flow hood should be cleaned top to bottom front to back, with a disinfectant solution.
   a. True
   b. False

3. The syringe plunger can be removed from the barrel before use.
   a. True
   b. False

4. List three points of the underlying principle of the laminar flow hood:

   _____

   _____

   _____

   _____

5. What is the purpose of alternating cleansers?

   _____

   _____

   _____

   _____

Please return to the videotape.

SECTION TWO: INTRODUCTION TO RISK LEVEL CLASSIFICATION

OVERVIEW

The ASHP TAB on "Quality Assurance for Pharmacy-Prepared Sterile Products" was developed on a concept of risk level related to patient outcome. When preparing sterile products, it is important to have a clear concept of what risk level a particular product falls into, and the condition and procedures under which that product should be prepared. This section will outline the parameters that should be used to determine risk level.

OBJECTIVES

Upon completion of this section, you should be able to:

- Name the three characteristics all compounded sterile products exhibit to be classified in risk level 1.

- Explain the reasons why compounded sterile products in risk levels 2 and 3 should meet or exceed all of the quality assurance recommendations for risk level 1.

- Name the three potential characteristics that sterile products exhibit to be classified in risk level 2.

- Name the two characteristics that sterile products could exhibit to be classified in risk level 3.

- Classify, by risk level, commonly pharmacy-prepared sterile products.

ASHP Technical Assistance Bulletin (Abridged)

Sterile products are grouped into three levels of risk to the patient, increasing from least (level 1) to greatest (level 3) potential risk and having different associated quality assurance recommendations for product integrity and patient safety. This classification system should assist pharmacists in selecting which sterile product preparation procedures to use. Compounded sterile products in risk levels 2 and 3 should meet or exceed all of the quality assurance recommendations for risk level 1. When circumstances make risk level assignment unclear, recommendations for the higher risk level should prevail. Pharmacists must exercise their own professional judgment in deciding which risk level applies to a specific compounded sterile product or situation. Consideration should be given to factors that increase potential risk to the patient, such as multiple system breaks, compounding complexities, high-risk administration sites, immuno-compromised status of the patient, use of non sterile components, microbial growth potential of the finished sterile drug product, storage conditions, and circumstances such as time between compounding and initiation of administration. The following risk assignments, based on the expertise of knowledgeable practitioners, represent on logical arrangement in which pharmacists may evaluate risk. Pharmacists may construct alternative arrangements that could be supported on the basis of scientific information and professional judgment.

Risk level 1. Risk level 1 applies to compounded sterile products that exhibit characteristics 1, 2, and 3 stated below. All risk level 1 products should be prepared with sterile equipment (e.g., syringes, vials), sterile ingredients and solutions, and sterile contact surfaces for the final product. Of the three risk levels, risk level 1 necessitates the least amount of quality assurance. Risk level 1 includes the following:

1. Products

   A. Stored at room temperature (see the appendix for temperature definitions and completely administered within 28 hours from preparation; or

   B. Stored under refrigeration for 7 days or less before complete administration to a patient over a period not to exceed 24 hours (Table 1) or

   C. Frozen for 30 days or less before complete administration to a patient over a period not to exceed 24 hours.

2. Unpreserved sterile products prepared for administration to one patient, or batch-prepared products containing suitable preservatives prepared for administration to more than one patient.

3. Products prepared by closed-system aseptic transfer of sterile, nonpyrogenic, finished pharmaceuticals obtained from licensed manufacturers into sterile final containers (e.g., syringe, minibag, portable infusion-device cassette) obtained from licensed manufacturers.

Risk level 2. Risk level 2 sterile products exhibit characteristic 1,2, *or* 3 stated below. All risk level 2 products should be prepared with sterile equipment, sterile ingredients and solutions, and sterile contact surfaces for the final product and by using closed-system transfer methods. Risk level 2 includes the following:

1. Products stored beyond 7 days under refrigeration, or stored beyond 30 days frozen, or administered beyond 28 hours after preparation and storage at room temperature (Table 1).

2. Batch-prepared products without preservatives that are intended for use by more than one patient. (Note: Batch-prepared products without preservatives that will be administered to multiple patients carry a greater risk to the patients than products prepared for a single patient because of the potential effect of product contamination on the health and well-being of a larger patient group.)

3. Products compounded by combining multiple sterile ingredients, obtained from licensed manufacturers, in a sterile reservoir, obtained from a licensed manufacturer, by using closed-system aseptic transfer before subdivision into multiple units to be dispensed to patients.

Risk level 3. Risk level 3 products exhibit either characteristic 1 *or* 2:

1. Products compounded from non sterile ingredients or compounded with non sterile components, containers or equipment.

2. Products prepared by combining multiple ingredients-sterile or non sterile-by using an open-system transfer or open reservoir before terminal sterilization or subdivision into multiple units to be dispensed.

DISCUSSION POINTS

⊃ The risk level classification system is designed to assist a pharmacist in selecting which preparation procedures will help to ensure the maximum patient safety at the least possible consumption of resources.

⊃ Pharmacists should exercise professional judgement in deciding which risk level applies to the specific sterile product.

⊃ Please note that the risk level classification system and the ASHP TAB on "Quality Assurance for Pharmacy-Prepared Sterile Products" are not intended to apply to the manufacture of sterile products as defined by state and federal laws and regulations, nor do they apply to the preparation of medications by pharmacists, nurses, or physicians in emergency situations for immediate administration to patients.

⊃ Many factors contribute to increasing potential risk to patients who receive sterile products. Those factors include:
  • drug stability
  • multiple system breaks
  • compounding complexities

- high-risk administration sites
- immunocompromised status of the patient
- use of non-sterile components
- microbial growth potential of finished sterile product
- storage conditions
- time between compounding and medication administration

⊃ Pharmacists in different practice settings (e.g., institutional, home, and long term care) with different distances between patients and pharmacy and variants in time between contact with a pharmacist and the patient, may experience unexpected outcomes as a result of the factors listed above. It is imperative that risk level assignment and subsequent preparation procedures result in labeling with expiration dates that ensure a safe and effective product.

Table 1
Assignment of Products Risk Level 1 or 2 According to
Time and Temperature Before Completion of Administration

Risk Level	Room Temperature (15 to 30° C)	Days of Storage	
		Refrigerator (2 to 8° C)	Freezer (-20 to -10°C)
1	Completely administered within 28 hrs.	≥7	≤30
2	Storage and administration exceeds 28 hrs.	>7	>30

Table one lists the risk level, room temperature, and the days of storage for both refrigerator and freezer for the assignment of products to the respective categories.

Table 1

Risk Level Comparison Summary

Risk Level	Time of Storage including Administration Time	Temperature of Storage	Ingredient Characteristics	Preparation Characteristics
1	<28 hours <7 days <30 days	Room temp. Refrigerated Frozen	Unpreserved sterile product for single patient batch prepared with preservative.	Prepared closed system via sterile transfer devices into sterile final containers
2	>7 days >30 days >28 hours of administration	Refrigerated Frozen Room temp.	Batch prepared for use by more than ibe person.	Prepared closed system by combining multiple sterile ingredients using aseptic. transfer.
3	Any length of storage	Room or Refrigerated.or Frozen	Non-sterile ingredients or Non-sterile combined with sterile ingredients.	Non-sterile components, equipment, or combination of sterile and non-sterile before terminal sterilization.

Please review Table 2 at this time for a summary of the differences between risk levels 1 and 2. Many, if not most, of your products will be risk level 1 or 2.

Risk level 3 classification is for drug products compounded in your pharmacy from either nonsterile ingredients or compounded with nonsterile components, containers, or equipment. In addition, risk level 3 products are defined as products prepared by combining multiple ingredients—sterile or non sterile—by using an open-system transfer or open reservoir before terminal sterilization or subdivision into multiple units to be dispensed. Please note that all risk level 3 products must be terminally sterilized in some fashion before dispensing.

SUMMARY

The risk level classification system was developed to distinguish between various pharmacy prepared sterile products and their methods of preparation in order to maximize safety and minimize the work necessary to assure a quality product.

EXERCISES

1. Apply a risk level to the following common pharmacy prepared products:

Risk Level	Sterile Product	Storage Method	Storage Time
_____	Acetazolamide in 50 ml D5W	Refrigerated	24 hours
_____	Amphotericin B in 500 ml D5W	Refrigerated	24 hours
_____	Ampicillin 1gm in 50 ml N.S.	Refrigerated	24 hours
_____	Azathioprine 100mg in 100 mls N.S.	Refrigerated	24 hours
_____	Carbenicillin 5gm in 100 mls N.S.	Frozen	10 days
_____	Cefonicid 1gm in 100ml D5W	Frozen	20 days
_____	Cefoperazone 1gm in 50ml D5W	Refrigerated	24 hours
_____	Cefotxine 2gm in 100 ml D5W	Frozen	5 days
_____	Cimetedine 300mg in 50 mls D5W	Frozen (100 made)	10 days
_____	TPN	Refrigerated	10 days at home
_____	Solutions with added Mg Cl$_2$ crystals	Refrigerated	12 hours
_____	Talc powder	Refrigerated	7 days

2. From your own pharmacy, make a list of the 10 most commonly prepared sterile products. Place them in the appropriate risk levels.

_____

_____

_____

_____

3. From your completed list in exercise 2 above, indicate why the prepared sterile products are placed in the respective risk level.

_____

_____

_____

_____

4. List all products made in your pharmacy that are risk level 3.

_____

_____

_____

_____

SELF-ASSESSMENT QUESTIONS

1. Batch prepared, frozen antibiotics using a closed system that are stored less than 14 days are risk level 1 products.

   a. True
   b. False

2. Non-sterile ingredients may classify a product to be risk level 2.

   a. True
   b. False

3. Most pharmacy prepared products will be classified as risk level 3.
   a. True
   b. False

4. Risk level 3 classification is for drugs compounded in your pharmacy from either sterile ingredients or compounded with nonsterile components, container, or equipment.
   a. True
   b. False

5. The primary difference between risk level 1 and 2 is the amount of administration and/or storage time of a sterile product.
   a. True
   b. False

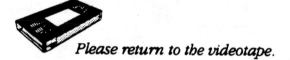

Please return to the videotape.

SECTION THREE: QUALITY ASSURANCE FOR RISK LEVEL ONE

OVERVIEW

As you reviewed earlier, the ASHP TAB separates risk levels into three categories. As you have learned, most of the products you prepare will fall into risk level 1. This section of your workbook will provide you with an in-depth discussion of the elements identifying risk level 1.

OBJECTIVES

Upon completion of this section, you should be able to:

- Describe the contents of well written policies and procedures for compounding sterile products in risk level 1.

- Identify personnel training requirements for preparing products in risk level 1.

- Practice proper storage and handling requirements in accordance with manufacturer or USP requirements.

- Identify the clean room requirements for risk level 1.

- Practice proper hygienic procedures when preparing sterile products.

- Describe why process validation is important and how to conduct process simulation testing.

- Employ a system that establishes proper assignment of substance expiration dates and identify sources of drug stability information.

- Employ proper labeling guidelines for a prescription or medication order.

- Recognize product or container deficiency by an end-product evaluation.

- Conduct a systematic approach to essential documentation.

3.1 ASHP Technical Assistance Bulletin (Abridged)

Quality assurance for risk level 1

RL 1.1: Policies and procedures.

Up-to-date policies and procedures for compounding sterile products should be written and available to all personnel involved in these activities. Policies and procedures should be reviewed at least annually by the designated pharmacist and department head and updated, as necessary, to reflect current standards of practice and quality. Additions, revisions, and deletions should be communicated to all personnel involved in sterile compounding and related activities. These policies and procedures should address personnel education and training requirements, competency evaluation, product acquisition, storage and handling of products and supplies, storage and delivery of final products, use and maintenance of facilities and equipment, appropriate garb and conduct for personnel working in the controlled area, process validation, preparation, technique, labeling, documentation, and quality control. Further, written policies and procedures should address personnel access and movement of materials into and near the controlled area. Policies and procedures for monitoring environmental conditions in the controlled area should take into consideration the amount of exposure of the product to the environment during compounding. Before compounding sterile products, all personnel involved should read the policies and procedures and sign to verify their understanding.

RL 1.2: Personnel education, training, and evaluation.

Pharmacy personnel preparing or dispensing sterile products should receive suitable didactic and experiential training and competency evaluation through demonstration testing (written or practical), or both. Some aspects that should be included in training programs include aseptic technique; critical-area contamination factors; environmental monitoring; facilities, equipment, and supplies; sterile product calculations and terminology; sterile product compounding documentation; quality assurance procedures; aseptic preparation procedures; proper gowning and gloving technique; and general conduct in the controlled area. In addition to knowledge of chemical, pharmaceutical, and clinical properties of drugs, pharmacists should also be knowledgeable about the principles of Current Good Manufacturing Practices. Videotapes and additional information on the essential components of a training, orientation, and evaluation program are described elsewhere. All pharmacy personnel involved in cleaning and maintenance of the controlled area should be knowledgeable about cleanroom design (if applicable), the basic concepts of aseptic compounding, and critical-area contamination factors. Non pharmacy personnel (e.g., housekeeping staff) involved in the cleaning or maintenance of the controlled area should receive adequate training on applicable procedures.

The aseptic technique of each person preparing sterile products should be observed and evaluated as satisfactory during orientation and training and at least on an annual basis thereafter. In addition to observation, methods of evaluating the knowledge of personnel include written or practical tests and process validation.

DISCUSSION POINTS

Please read the preceding ASHP TAB 3.1 before you continue.

3.1 Policies, Procedures, and Personnel Training Programs

It is sometimes difficult to know how to start documenting and implementing policies and procedures for the workplace. Included below are some examples of quality assurance policies and procedures and training programs that could be used as a template to customize for your own working environment. Please take a moment to look these over.

You can refer to these checklists for guidance when compiling your own documents.

RL 1.1: Policies and procedures

◊ personnel education and training requirements

◊ competency evaluation

◊ product acquisition

◊ storage and handling of products and supplies

◊ storage and delivery of final products

◊ use and maintenance of facilities and equipment

◊ appropriate garb and conduct for personnel working in controlled area

◊ process validation

◊ preparation technique

◊ labeling

◊ documentation

◊ quality control

RL 1.2: Personnel training programs

◊ aseptic technique

◊ critical-area contamination factors

◊ environmental monitoring

◊ facilities, equipment, and supplies

◊ sterile product calculations and terminology

◊ sterile product compounding documentation

◊ quality assurance procedures

◊ aseptic preparation procedures

◊ proper gowning and gloving technique

◊ general conduct in the controlled area

◊ principles of "Current Good Manufacturing Practices"

◊ cleanroom design

◊ basic concepts of aseptic compounding

◊ critical-area contamination factors

Please return to the videotape.

3.2 ASHP Technical Assistance Bulletin (Abridged)

RL 1.3: Storage and handling. Solutions, drugs, supplies, and equipment used to prepare or administer sterile products should be stored in accordance with manufacturer or USP requirements. Temperatures in refrigerators and freezers used to store ingredients and finished sterile preparations should be monitored and documented daily to ensure that compendial storage requirements are met. Warehouse and other pharmacy storage areas where ingredients are stored should be monitored to ensure that temperature, light, moisture, and ventilation remain within manufacturer and compendial requirements. To permit adequate floor cleaning, drugs and supplies should be stored on shelving areas above the floor. Products that have exceeded their expiration dates should be removed from active storage areas. Before use, each drug, ingredient, and container should be visually inspected for damage, defects, and expiration date.

Unnecessary personnel traffic in the controlled area should be minimized. Particle-generating activities, such as removal of intravenous solutions, drug, and supplies from cardboard boxes, should not be performed in the controlled area. Products and supplies used in preparing sterile products should be removed from shipping containers outside the controlled area before aseptic processing is begun. Packaging materials and items generating unacceptable amounts of particles (e.g., cardboard boxes, paper towels, reference books) should not be permitted in the controlled area or critical area. The removal of immediate packaging designed to retain the sterility or stability of a product (e.g., syringe packaging, light-resistant pouches) is an exception; obviously, this type of packaging should not be removed outside the controlled area. Disposal of packaging materials, used syringes, containers, and needles should be performed at least daily, and more often if needed, to enhance sanitation and avoid accumulation in the controlled area.

In the event of a product recall, there should be a mechanism for tracking and retrieving affected products from specific patients to whom the products were dispensed.

RL 1.4: Facilities and equipment. The controlled area should be a limited-access area sufficiently separated from other pharmacy operations to minimize the potential for contamination that could result from the unnecessary flow of materials and personnel into and out of the area. Computer entry, order processing, label generation, and record keeping should be performed outside the critical area. The controlled area should be clean, well lighted, and of sufficient size to support sterile compounding activities. For hand washing, a sink with hot and cold running water should be in close proximity. Refrigeration, freezing, ventilation, and room temperature control capabilities appropriate for storage of ingredients, supplies, and pharmacy-prepared sterile products in accordance with manufacturer, USP, and state or federal requirements should exist. The controlled area should be cleaned and disinfected at regular intervals with appropriate agents, according to written policies and procedures. Disinfectants should be alternated periodically to prevent the development of resistant microorganisms. The floors of the controlled area should be nonporous and washable to enable regular disinfection. Active work surfaces in the controlled area (e.g., carts, compounding devices, counter surfaces) should be disinfected, in accordance with written procedures. Refrigerators, freezers, shelves, and other areas where pharmacy-prepared sterile products are stored should be kept clean.

Sterile products should be prepared in a Class 100 environment. Such an environment exists inside a certified horizontal- or vertical-laminar-airflow hood. Facilities that meet the recommendations for risk level 3 preparation would be suitable for risk level 1 and 2 compounding. Cytotoxic and other hazardous products should be prepared in a Class II biological-safety cabinet. Laminar-airflow hoods are designed to be operated continuously. If a laminar-airflow hood is turned off between aseptic processing, it should be operated long enough to allow complete purging of room air from the critical area (e.g., 15-30 minutes), then disinfected before use. The critical-area work surface and all accessible interior surfaces of the hood should be disinfected with an appropriate agent before work begins and periodically thereafter, in accordance with written policies and procedures. The exterior surfaces of the laminar-airflow hood should be cleaned periodically with a mild detergent or suitable disinfectant; 70% isopropyl alcohol may damage the hood's clear plastic surfaces. The laminar-airflow hood should be certified by a qualified contractor at least every six months or when it is relocated to ensure operational efficiency and integrity.

Prefilters in the laminar-air-flow hood should be changed periodically, in accordance with written policies and procedures. A method should be established to calibrate and verify the accuracy of automated compounding devices used in aseptic processing.

RL 1.5 Garb. Procedures should generally require that personnel wear clean clothing covers that generate low amounts of particles in the controlled area. Clean gowns or closed coats with sleeves that have elastic binding at the cuff are recommended. Hand, finger, and wrist jewelry should be minimized or eliminated. Head and facial hair should be covered. Masks are recommended during aseptic preparation procedures.

Personnel preparing sterile products should scrub their hands and arms (to the elbow) with an appropriate antimicrobial skin cleanser.

DISCUSSION POINTS

Please read the preceding ASHP TAB 3.2 before you continue.

3.2 Storage and Handling, Facilities and Equipment, Garb

The following is a summary of quality assurance recommendations that should be considered in the handling of sterile products:

RL 1.3: Storage and handling

◊ solutions, drugs, supplies, and equipment used to prepare or administer sterile products should be stored in accordance with manufacturer or USP requirements.

◊ refrigerator and freezer temperatures should be monitored and documented daily to meet compendial storage requirements.

◊ storage areas were ingredients are stored should be monitored to ensure temperature, light, moisture, and ventilation remain within manufacturer and compendial requirements.

◊ drugs and supplies should be stored on shelving areas above floor.

◊ remove all products that have exceeded their expiration dates.

◊ inspect each drug, ingredient and container for damage, defects and expiration date.

◊ keep unnecessary personnel traffic in controlled area to minimum.

◊ packaging of materials and items generating unacceptable amounts of particles should not be permitted in controlled area.

◊ keep controlled area sanitary by daily disposals of used syringes, containers, and needles.

◊ initiate system for tracking and retrieving recalled products from patients to whom they were dispensed.

The bulk storage of small volume injections and large volume parenterals and many other drugs requires boxes, cartons and cases of paper and plastic materials. These materials will shed particles when they are opened and unpacked. This shedding is a controllable function that must be done away from the sterile products area.

RL 1.4: Facilities and equipment

◊ controlled area should have limited access and be separated from other pharmacy operations.

◊ controlled area should be clean, well lighted, and of sufficient size to support sterile compounding activities.

◊ clean and disinfect controlled areas at regular intervals including refrigerators, freezers and shelves where products are stored.

◊ a sink should be located nearby for hand washing.

◊ sterile products should be prepared in a Class 100 environment.

◊ prepare all cytotoxic and other hazardous products in a Class II biological-safety cabinet or vertical hood environment.

◊ the exterior surfaces of the laminar-airflow hood should be cleaned periodically with a mild detergent or suitable disinfectant.

The controlled area is the clean room or room in which the sterile products are prepared in a laminar flow hood. For risk level 1 products, no specific monitoring of air particles or air borne microbial contaminates is suggested. This recommendation will change as we progress to risk level 2. It is recommended that the controlled area is separate from the rest of the pharmacy operation to minimize contamination and distraction of employees.

RL 1.5: Garb

◊ personnel should wear clean clothing covers that generate low amounts of particles in the controlled area.

◊ cover your head and facial hair and wear a mask during all aseptic preparation procedures.

◊ scrub to the elbow with an appropriate anti microbial skin cleanser.

Contaminated hands are a very frequent source of microbial contamination. Therefore, persons working in a pharmacy should frequently wash their hands during the work day with a suitable antimicrobial skin cleanser. This point should be continually stressed to all employees.

EXERCISES

In order to complete these exercises, you should have the following materials available:

* temperature logs for refrigerator
* your institution's hand washing policy
* your institution's procedures for cleaning the controlled area

1. For your pharmacy operation list the 5 most commonly used drugs that must be opened or unpacked outside the controlled area.

    _____

    _____

    _____

    _____

2. Review the temperature logs for your refrigerator for the past 60 days. List any variations outside the ranges and what was done to correct the situation.

    _____

    _____

    _____

    _____

3. Review your pharmacy's policy on hand washing. Are you using the correct antimicrobial?

    _____

    _____

    _____

    _____

4. Review the procedures for cleaning the controlled area of your pharmacy.

SELF-ASSESSMENT QUESTIONS

1. The USP has limits and definitions of temperature requirements for refrigeration and freezing.
   a. True
   b. False

2. Light resistant packaging for light sensitive drugs must be removed before taking into the controlled area.
   a. True
   b. False

3. The controlled room housing the laminar flow hood should be separated from the pharmacy dispensing area.
   a. True
   b. False

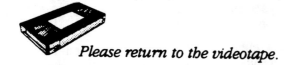

Please return to the videotape.

3.3–3.4 ASHP Technical Assistance Bulletin (Abridged)

RL 1.6: Aseptic technique and product preparation. Sterile products should be prepared with aseptic technique in a Class 100 environment. Personnel should scrub their hands and forearms for an appropriate length of time with a suitable antimicrobial skin cleanser at the beginning of each aseptic compounding process and when re-entering the controlled area. Personnel should wear appropriate attire (see RL 1.5: Garb). Eating, drinking, and smoking should be prohibited in the controlled area. Talking should be minimized in the critical area during aseptic preparation.

Ingredients used to compound sterile products should be determined to be stable, compatible, and appropriate for the product to be prepared, according to manufacturer or USP guidelines or appropriate scientific references. The ingredients of the preparation should be predetermined to be suitable to result in a final product that meets physiological norms for solution osmolality and pH, as appropriate for the intended route of administration. Each ingredient and container should be inspected for defects, expiration date, and product integrity before use. Expired, inappropriately stored, or defective products should not be used in preparing sterile products. Defective products should be promptly reported to the FDA.

Only materials essential for preparing the sterile product should be placed in the laminar-airflow hood. The surfaces of ampuls, vials, and container closures (e.g., vial stoppers) should be disinfected by swabbing or spraying with an appropriate disinfectant solution (e.g., 70% isopropyl alcohol) before placement in the hood. Materials used in aseptic preparation should be arranged in the critical area of the hood in a manner that prevents interruption of the unidirectional airflow between the high-efficiency particulate air (HEPA) filter and critical sites of needles, vials, ampuls, containers, and transfer sets. All aseptic procedures should be performed at least 6 inches inside the front edge of the laminar-airflow hood, in a clear path of unidirectional airflow between the HEPA filter and work materials (e.g., needles, stoppers). The number of personnel preparing sterile products in the hood at one time should be minimized. Overcrowding of the critical work area may interfere with unidirectional airflow and increase the potential for compounding errors. Likewise, the number of units being prepared in the hood at one time should be consistent with the amount of work space in the critical area. Automated compounding devices and other equipment placed in or adjacent to the critical area should be cleaned, disinfected, and placed to avoid contamination or disruption of the unidirectional airflow between the HEPA filter and sterile surfaces.

Aseptic technique should be used to avoid touch contamination of sterile needles, syringe parts (e.g., plunger, syringe tip), and other critical sites. Solutions from ampuls should be properly filtered to remove particles. Solutions of reconstituted powders should be mixed carefully, ensuring complete dissolution of the drug with the appropriate diluent. Needle entry into vials with rubber stoppers should be done cautiously to avoid the creation of rubber core particles. Before, during, and after the preparation of sterile products, the pharmacist should carefully check the identity and verify the amounts of the ingredients in sterile preparations against the original prescription, medication order, or other appropriate documentation (e.g., computerized patient profile, label generated from a pharmacist-verified order) before the product is released or dispensed. Additional information on aseptic technique is available elsewhere.

For preparation involving automated compounding devices, data entered into the compounding device should be verified by a pharmacist before compounding begins and end-product checks should be performed to verify accuracy of ingredient delivery. These checks may include weighing and visually verifying the final product. For example, the expected weight (in grams) of the final product, based on the specific gravities of the ingredients and their respective volumes, can be documented on the compounding formula sheet, dated, and initialed by the responsible pharmacist. Once compounding is completed, each final product can be weighed and its weight compared with the expected weight. The product's actual weight should fall within a pre-established threshold for variance. Visual verification may be aided by marking the beginning level of each bulk container before starting the automated mixing process and checking each container after completing the mixing process to determine whether the final levels appear reasonable in comparison with expected volumes. The operator should also periodically observe the device during the mixing process to ensure that the device is operating properly (e.g., check to see that all stations are operating). If there are doubts whether a product or component has been properly prepared or stored, then the product should not be used. Refractive index measurements may also be used to verify the addition of certain ingredients.

RL 1.7: Process validation. Validation of aseptic processing procedures provides a mechanism for ensuring that processes consistently result in sterile products of acceptable quality. For most aseptic preparation procedures, process validation is actually a method of assessing the adequacy of a person's aseptic technique. It is recommended that each individual involved in the preparation of sterile products successfully complete a validation process on technique before being allowed to prepare sterile products. The validation process should follow a written procedure that includes evaluation of technique through process simulation.

Process simulation testing is valuable for assessing the compounding process, especially aseptic fill operations. It allows for the evaluation of opportunities for microbial contamination during all steps of sterile product preparation. The sterility of the final product is a cumulative function of all processes involved in its preparation and is ultimately determined by the processing step providing the lowest probability of sterility. Process simulation testing is carried out in the same manner as normal production except that an appropriate microbiological growth medium is used in place of the actual products used during sterile preparation. The growth medium is processed as if it were a product being compounded for patient use; the same personnel, procedures, equipment, and materials are involved. The medium samples are then incubated and evaluated. If no microbial growth is detected, this provides evidence that adequate aseptic technique was used. If growth is detected, the entire sterile preparation process must be evaluated, corrective action taken, and the process simulation test performed again. No products intended for patient use should be prepared by an individual until the process simulation test indicates that the individual can competently perform aseptic procedures. It is recommended that personnel competency be revalidated at least annually, whenever the quality assurance program yields an unacceptable result, and whenever unacceptable techniques are observed; this revalidation should be documented.

DISCUSSION POINTS

Please read the preceding ASHP TAB 3.3–3.4 before you continue.

3.3 Aseptic Technique and Product Preparation

Please review the information presented in Section One of this program entitled, "Aseptic Preparation of Parenteral Products". Understanding the information will provide the building block for aseptic technique and product preparation for risk level 1 products. Please review again the specific paragraphs of the ASHP TAB discussing risk level 1. Listed below are several important points to consider when preparing sterile products.

RL 1.6: Aseptic technique and product preparation

◊ all aseptic procedures should be performed at least 6 inches inside the laminar-airflow hood.

◊ do not overcrowd the critical work area.

◊ make sure the number of units is consistent with amount of work space in critical area.

◊ only essential materials should be placed in the laminar flow hood.

◊ all ingredients should be stable, compatible and appropriate for product that is being prepared.

◊ do not use expired, inappropriately stored or defective products when preparing sterile products.

◊ when using automated compounding devices for preparation, verify data entered by pharmacist.

3.4 Process Validation

Risk level 1 recommendations concerning process validation, in practice, constitute a method of assessing the adequacy of a person's aseptic technique.

Process simulation testing is valuable for:

- assessing the compounding process

- evaluating the opportunities for microbial contamination during all steps of sterile product preparation.

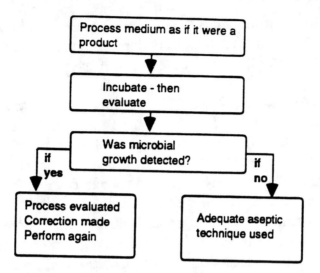

This testing is carried out in the same manner as normal production except that an appropriate microbiological growth medium is used in place of the actual products used during sterile preparation.

TIPS

➤ If microbial growth is detected, have any organisms that have grown identified. Knowing the identity of the organism will give you a clue to its source. For example, staphylococcus might indicate touch contamination from poor aseptic technique, while a fungus would more likely be associated with environmental contamination, such as an unclean hood.

➤ If a breakdown in aseptic technique is found with more than one employee, review your training procedures; this may indicate a problem in your department's training program, rather than simply employee technique.

EXERCISES

In order to complete these exercises, you should have the following materials available:

✳ commercially available aseptic technique testing device
✳ your institution's policies and procedures for aseptic technique

1. Using an ATTACK™ kit or other commercially available aseptic technique testing device, demonstrate the transfer of a liquid drug and the constitution and transfer of a sterile powder. First withdraw a suitable amount of fluid from a vial containing trypticase soy broth (TSB) and transfer this to an empty sterile vial. Incubate this vial for 10-14 days and observe for microbial growth. Next, withdraw a suitable amount of fluid from a vial containing TSB and transfer this into a vial containing soluble, chemically inactive powder. Shake or swirl the vial gently until the powder is completely dissolved. Withdraw a suitable amount of this solution and transfer it to an empty sterile vial. Incubate this vial for 10–14 days and observe for microbial growth. Should either vial exhibit growth, review the section of the videotape and workbook on aseptic technique and repeat this exercise.

2. Review your pharmacy's policies and procedures for aseptic techniques. Do they conform to the recommendations presented here? If they are different, why is that the case?

    _____

    _____

    _____

    _____

SELF-ASSESSMENT QUESTIONS

1. The purpose of process validation is:
    a. to verify the aseptic technique of the preparer.
    b. to assure the procedure will produce a sterile product every time.
    c. all of the above.
    d. none of the above.

2. Process simulation testing duplicates the procedure of preparing a sterile product, but substitutes the constituents of the sterile product with:

    a. sterile water

    b. micro biological growth media

    c. sample microorganisms

    d. normal saline

3. A positive result, or growth of a microorganism, in process simulation testing might indicate:

    a. poor aseptic technique

    b. environmental contamination

    c. a breakdown in the process

    d. a. and b.

    e. all of the above

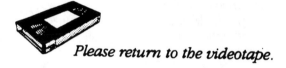

Please return to the videotape.

3.5 ASHP Technical Assistance Bulletin (Abridged)

RL 1.8: Expiration dating. All pharmacy-prepared sterile products should bear an appropriate expiration date. The expiration date assigned should be based on currently available drug stability information and sterility considerations. Sources of drug stability information include references (e.g., *Remington's Pharmaceutical Sciences, Handbook on Injectable Drugs*), manufacturer recommendations, and reliable, published research. When interpreting published drug stability information, the pharmacist should consider all aspects of the final sterile product being prepared (e.g., drug reservoir, drug concentration, storage conditions). Methods used for establishing expiration dates should be documented. Appropriate inhouse (or contract service) stability testing may be used to determine expiration dates.

RL 1.9: Labeling. Sterile products should be labeled with at least the following information:

1. For patient-specific products: the patient's name and any other appropriate patient identification (e.g., location, identification number); for batch-prepared products: control or lot number;

2. All solution and ingredient names, amounts, strengths, and concentrations (when applicable);

3. Expiration date (and time, when applicable);

4. Prescribed administration regimen, when appropriate (including rate and route of administration);

5. Appropriate auxiliary labeling (including precautions);

6. Storage requirements;

7. Identification (e.g., initials) of the responsible pharmacist;

8. Device-specific instructions (when appropriate); and

9. Any additional information, in accordance with state or federal requirements.

It may also be useful to include a reference number for the prescription or medication order in the labeling; this information is usually required for products dispensed to outpatients. The label should be legible and affixed to the final container in a manner enabling it to be read while the sterile product is being administered (when possible).

RL 1.10: End-product evaluation. The final product should be inspected and evaluated for container leaks, container integrity, solution cloudiness, particulates in the solution, appropriate solution color, and solution volume when preparation is completed and again when the product is dispensed. The responsible pharmacist should verify that the product was compounded accurately with respect to the

use of correct ingredients, quantities, containers, and reservoirs; different methods may be used for end-product verification (e.g., observation, calculation checks, documented records).

RL 1.11: Documentation. The following should be documented and maintained on file for an adequate period of time, according to organizational policies and procedures and state regulatory requirements: (1) the training and competency evaluation of employees in sterile product procedures, (2) refrigerator and freezer temperatures, and (3) certification of laminar-airflow hoods. Pharmacists should also maintain appropriate dispensing records for sterile products, in accordance with state regulatory requirements.

DISCUSSION POINTS

Please read the preceding ASHP TAB 3.5 before you continue.

3.5 Expiration Dating, Labeling, End-product Evaluation, Documentation

The next several sections deal directly with the prepared sterile product. Proper **expiration dating** is vital, since dispensing of an expired drug product could lead to administration of a sub-therapeutic dose of medication. **Labeling** is of critical importance, because the label provides the direct link between the physician's order and the product-in-hand. The label should allow for verification of such items as correct patient, drug, dose, rate and route of administration, expiration date, and lot number in the event of a product recall. **End-product evaluation** is a simple visual inspection of the finished product and review of its preparation procedure which ensures that patients are getting safe, accurate dosage forms. Finally, **documentation** provides written records of the competence of personnel and the fitness of preparation and storage equipment. This documentation is often required by JCAHO and other accrediting organizations. Refer to the following bulleted lists for a summary on these subjects.

RL 1.8: Expiration dating

◊ assigning an expiration date to a pharmacy-prepared sterile product should be done following an established procedure yet easy to implement and follow.

◊ evaluation of expiration dates should be done on a product by product basis and be based on currently available drug stability information and sterility considerations.

◊ when interpreting this information, consider all aspects of final sterile product such as *drug reservoir, drug concentration, storage conditions.*

◊ methods for establishing expiration dates should be documented.

◊ appropriate in-house (or contract service) stability testing may be used to determine expiration dates.

RL 1.9: Labeling

Remember to label sterile products with at least the following:

◊ patient name and identification (if patient-specific)

◊ control of lot number (if batch- prepared)

◊ all solution & ingredient names, amounts, strengths, and concentrations

◊ expiration date and time

◊ prescribed administration regimen including rate and route

◊ appropriate auxiliary labeling

◊ storage requirements

◊ identification of pharmacist

◊ device-specific instructions

◊ state of federal information

RL 1.10: End-product evaluation

The final product should be inspected for:

◊ container leaks

◊ container integrity

◊ solution cloudiness

◊ particulates in the solution

◊ appropriate solution color

◊ solution volume when preparation is completed product dispensed

◊ verification that product was compounded accurately

Risk level one standards state that the following should be properly documented and maintained on file for a specified period of time:

RL 1.11: Documentation

◊ training and competency evaluation of employees in sterile product procedures

◊ refrigerator and freezer temperatures

◊ certification of laminar-airflow hoods

◊ dispensing records for sterile products, in accordance with state regulatory requirements

---

SUMMARY

The classification of pharmacy-prepared sterile-products can fall into three risk level categories. Regardless of the risk level, an organized approach to quality assurance must be taken. This quality assurance program must address at least the following: policies and procedures; personnel education, training, and evaluation; storage and handling; facilities and equipment; garb; aseptic technique and product preparation; process validation; expiration dating; and documentation.

The quality assurance guidelines outlined here for risk level 1, will encompass the majority of pharmacy-prepared sterile products.

TIPS

➤ To avoid disastrous confusion, add some type of prefix or suffix to expiration dates to indicate whether they represent frozen, refrigerated, or room temperature expiration. (Example: R04/12/94 for a product that expires on April 12, 1994 under refrigeration.)

➤ To help you remember to perform a thorough end-product evaluation, be sure to CLIP each product prepared:

- **C**olor and clarity of the solution
- **L**eaks from the container
- **I**ntegrity of the container
- **P**articulates in the solution

EXERCISES

In order to complete these exercises, you should have the following materials available:

* records on training and equipment integrity

1. Review your department's expiration dating policy. Is there a standard process developed for determining expiration dates? If not, determine how expiration dates are assigned.

2. Review any records your department currently keeps on training and equipment integrity. Develop a sign-off sheet for documentation of refrigerator/freezer temperatures and hood cleanings.

SELF-ASSESSMENT QUESTIONS

1. When determining an expiration date for a pharmacy prepared sterile product, you must consider the
    a. drug reservoir
    b. diluent and/or vehicle
    c. drug concentration
    d. storage conditions
    e. all of the above

2. The product expiration date and time does not have to appear on the label if the product was patient-specific.
    a. True
    b. False

3. The control or lot number that must appear on the label of batch prepared sterile products is:
    a. an internal lot number indicating the date of preparation and referring back to a compounding log.
    b. the manufacturer's lot number for the ingredient drug being prepared.

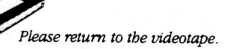

Please return to the videotape.

SECTION FOUR: QUALITY ASSURANCE FOR RISK LEVEL TWO

OVERVIEW

In Section Three, you reviewed the quality assurance guidelines that should be met for risk level one. In this section, you will learn what end-product qualities separate risk level one and risk level two classification.

OBJECTIVES

Upon completion of this section, you should be able to:

- Describe why stringent requirements are required for risk level 2 preparation.

- Describe risk level 1 policies and procedures and identify and define necessary environmental monitoring devices and techniques to be used to ensure an adequate environment for risk level 2 sterile product preparation.

- Identify personnel requirements for preparing products specific to risk level 2.

- Practice proper storage and handling requirements in accordance with manufacturer or USP requirements.

- Identify the clean room requirements for risk level 1 and list five additional recommendations specific to risk level 2 sterile product preparation.

- Practice proper hygienic procedures when preparing sterile products to include use of gloves, gowns, masks and shoe covers.

- Describe risk level 1 aseptic technique and product preparation and describe a system for monitoring preparation of batch sterile products specific to risk level 2.

- Describe why process validation is important and how to conduct process simulation testing for risk level 2 sterile products.

- Employ a system that establishes proper assignment of product expiration dates and identify sources of drug stability information.

- Employ proper labeling guidelines for a prescription or medication order.

- Recognize product or container deficiency by an end-product evaluation and, specific to risk level 2, conduct end-product sterility testing according to a formal sampling plan.

- Conduct a systematic approach to essential documentation to include end-product sampling and batch-preparation records specific to risk level 2 sterile products.

4.1–4.2 ASHP Technical Assistance Bulletin (Abridged)

Because the risks associated with contamination of a sterile product are increased with long-term storage and administration, more stringent requirements are appropriate for risk level 2 preparation.

RL 2.1: Policies and procedures. In addition to all recommendations for risk level 1, the written quality assurance program should define and identify necessary environmental monitoring devices and techniques to be used to ensure an adequate environment for risk level 2 sterile product preparation. Examples include the use of airborne particle counters, air velocity and temperature meters, viable particle samplers (e.g., slit samplers), agar plates, and swab sampling of surfaces and potential contamination sites. All aspects of risk level 2 sterile product preparation, storage, and distribution, including details such as the choice of cleaning materials and disinfectants and the monitoring of equipment accuracy, should be addressed in written policies and procedures. Limits of acceptability (threshold or action levels) for environmental monitoring and process simula-

tion and actions to be implemented when thresholds are exceeded should be defined in written policies. For sterile batch compounding, written policies and procedures should be established for the use of master formulas and work sheets and for appropriate documentation. Policies and procedures should also address personnel attire in the controlled area, lot number determination and documentation, and any other quality assurance procedures unique to compounding risk level 2 sterile products.

RL 2.2: Personnel education, training, and evaluation. All recommendations for risk level 1 should be met. In addition to recommendations for risk level 1, assessment of the competency of personnel preparing risk level 2 sterile products should include an appropriate process simulation procedure (as described in RL 1.7: Process validation). However, process simulation procedures for assessing the preparation of risk level 2 sterile products should be representative of all types of manipulations, products, and batch sizes personnel preparing risk level 2 products are likely to encounter.

RL 2.3: Storage and handling. All storage and handling recommendations for risk level 1 should be met.

RL 2.4: Facilities and equipment. In addition to all recommendations for risk level 1, the following are recommended for risk level 2 sterile product preparation:

1. Risk level 2 products should be prepared in a Class 100 horizontal- or vertical-laminar-airflow hood that is properly situated in a controlled area that meets Class 100,000 conditions (or better) for acceptable airborne particle levels. Class 100,000 conditions mean that no more than 100,000 particles 0.5 mm and larger may exist per cubic foot of air. A positive pressure relative to adjacent pharmacy areas is recommended.

2. Cleaning materials (e.g., mops, sponges, germicidal disinfectants) for use in the controlled area or clean-room should be carefully selected. They should be made of materials that generate a low amount of particles. If reused, cleaning materials should be cleaned and disinfected between uses.

3. The critical-area work surfaces (e.g., interior of the laminar-airflow hood) should be disinfected frequently and before and after each batch preparation process with an appropriate agent, according to written policies and procedures. Floors should be disinfected at least daily. Carpet or porous floors, porous walls, and porous ceiling tiles are not desirable in the controlled area because these surfaces cannot be properly disinfected. Exterior hood surfaces and other hard surfaces in the controlled area, such as shelves, carts, tables, and stools, should be disinfected weekly and after any unanticipated event that could increase the risk of contamination. Walls should be cleaned at least monthly.

4. To ensure that an appropriate environment is maintained for risk level 2 sterile product preparation, an effective written environmental monitoring program is recommended. Sampling of air and surfaces according to a written plan and schedule is recommended. The plan and frequency should be adequate to document that the controlled area is suitable and that the laminar-airflow hood(s) or biological-safety cabinet(s) meet the Class 100 requirements. Limits of acceptability (thresholds or action levels) and appropriate actions to be taken in the event thresholds are exceeded should be specified.

5. To help reduce the number of particles in the controlled area, an adjacent support area (e.g., anteroom) of high cleanliness, separated from the controlled area by a barrier (e.g., plastic curtain, partition, wall), is desirable. Appropriate activities for the support area include, but are not limited to, hand washing, gowning and gloving, removal of packaging and cardboard items, and cleaning and disinfecting hard-surface containers and supplies before placing these items in the controlled area.

RL 2.5: Garb. All recommendations for risk level 1 should be met. Gloves, gowns, and masks are recommended for the preparation of all risk level 2 sterile products. It must be emphasized that, even if sterile gloves are used, gloves do not remain sterile during aseptic compounding; however, they do assist in containing bacteria, skin, and other particles that may be shed, even from scrubbed hands. Clean gowns, coveralls, or closed jackets with sleeves having elastic binding at the cuff are recommended; these garments should be made of low-shedding materials. Shoe covers may be helpful in maintaining the cleanliness of the controlled area. During sterile product preparation, gloves should be rinsed frequently with a suitable agent (e.g., 70% isopropyl alcohol) and changed when their integrity is compromised (i.e., when they are punctured or torn).

DISCUSSION POINTS

Please read the preceding ASHP TAB 4.1–4.2 before you continue.

4.1 Policies and Procedures, Personnel Education, Training and Evaluation

Each risk level builds on the previous one. The difference between risk level one and risk level two is that the risks associated with contamination of a sterile products are increased with *long-term storage* and *administration*. Therefore more stringent requirements are needed for risk level two product preparation. Please review each of the following quality assurance summaries, taking note of how risk level 2 (noted in **bold** print) builds on risk level 1.

RL 2.1: Policies and procedures

◊ personnel education and training requirements
◊ competency evaluation
◊ product acquisition
◊ storage and handling of products and supplies
◊ storage and delivery of final products
◊ use and maintenance of facilities and equipment
◊ appropriate garb and conduct for personnel working in controlled area
◊ process validation
◊ preparation technique
◊ labeling
◊ documentation
◊ quality control

ADDITIONALLY...

◊ **define and identify necessary environmental monitoring devices and techniques such as air velocity, temperature meters, and agar plates.**

RL 2.2: Personnel education, training and evaluation

◊ aseptic technique
◊ critical-area contamination factors
◊ environmental monitoring
◊ facilities, equipment, and supplies
◊ sterile product calculations and terminology
◊ sterile product compounding documentation
◊ quality assurance procedures
◊ aseptic preparation procedures
◊ proper gowning and gloving technique
◊ general conduct in the controlled area
◊ principles of "Current Good Manufacturing Practices"
◊ cleanroom design
◊ basic concepts of aseptic compounding
◊ critical-area contamination factors

ADDITIONALLY...

◊ **periodically assess all personnel preparing risk level 2 products through appropriate process simulation procedure.**

4.2 Storage and Handling, Facilities and Equipment, Garb

Risk level 2 standards for storage and equipment are the same for risk level 1. However the recommended standards for facility and equipment and garb are more stringent.

RL 2.3: Storage and handling

◊ solutions, drugs, supplies, and equipment used to prepare or administer sterile products should be stored in accordance with manufacturer or USP requirements.

◊ refrigerator and freezer temperatures should be monitored and documented daily to meet compendial storage requirements.

◊ storage areas were ingredients are stored should be monitored to ensure temperature, light, moisture, and ventilation remain within manufacturer and compendial requirements.

◊ drugs and supplies should be stored on shelving areas above floor.

◊ remove all products that have exceeded their expiration dates

◊ inspect each drug, ingredient and container for damage, defects and expiration date.

◊ keep unnecessary personnel traffic in controlled area to minimum

◊ packaging of materials and items generating unacceptable amounts of particles should not be permitted in controlled area.

◊ keep controlled area sanitized by daily disposals of used syringes, containers, and needles.

◊ initiate system for tracking and retrieving affected products from patients to whom they were dispensed.

RL 2.4: Facilities and equipment

◊ controlled area should have limited access and be separated from other pharmacy operations.

◊ controlled area should be clean, well lighted, and of sufficient size to support sterile compounding activities.

◊ clean and disinfect controlled areas at regular intervals including refrigerators, freezers and shelves where products are stored.

◊ a sink should be located nearby for hand washing.

◊ prepare all cytotoxic and other hazardous products in a Class II biological-safety cabinet or vertical hood environment.

◊ the exterior surfaces of the laminar-airflow hood should be cleaned periodically with a mild detergent or suitable disinfectant.

ADDITIONALLY...

◊ *cleaning materials should be made of materials that generate a low amount of particles.*

◊ *create an adjacent support area of high cleanliness and separate with barrier*

◊ *the Class 100 critical area should be properly situated in a Class 100,000 controlled area.*

◊ *floors should be disinfected at least daily.*

◊ *external hood surfaces and other hard surfaces in the controlled area should be disinfected at least weekly. (This includes shelves, carts, and stools.)*

◊ *walls should be cleaned monthly.*

◊ *sampling of air and surfaces according to a written plan and schedule is recommended.*

RL 2.5: Garb

◊ personnel should wear clean clothing covers that generate low amounts of particles in the controlled area.

◊ cover your head and facial hair and wear a mask during all aseptic preparation procedures.

◊ scrub to the elbow with an appropriate anti microbial skin cleanser.

ADDITIONALLY...

◊ *gloves, gowns, masks and shoe covers are recommended.*

TIPS

➤ Place a cabinet/wardrobe in the anteroom near the entrance to the controlled area, which contains all necessary garb (gloves of various sizes, gowns, masks, head and shoe covers.) This keeps garb well-organized and prevents employees from forgetting all appropriate garb before entering the controlled area.

➤ Develop a calendar containing all appropriate quality control activities that need to be performed and the date to be completed (since some activities are daily, weekly, monthly, etc.). These might include checking refrigerator and freezer temperatures, cleaning hoods, cleaning controlled area carts or walls, etc. Display the calendar prominently.

EXERCISES

1. Prepare a daily checklist of environmental monitoring tasks. Be sure to include air and surface sampling as well as temperature and pressure measurements, and include established thresholds for each of these monitors for comparison with obtained values.

2. List 5 items/objects in the controlled area which would require periodic (i.e., weekly or monthly) cleaning.

_____

_____

_____

_____

SELF-ASSESSMENT QUESTIONS

1. Class 100,000 conditions mean that no more than 100,000 particles of this size or larger exist per cubic foot of air.

   a. 0.05 μm
   b. 0.1 μm
   c. 0.25 μm
   d. 0.5 μm

2. Gloves are not required in RL 2 compounding.

   a. True

   b. False

3. If a glove is punctured during batch preparation, it should:

   a. be replaced only when batch compounding is completed.

   b. be replaced immediately.

   c. be left on and used for remainder of day.

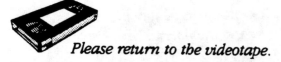

Please return to the videotape.

4.3–4.4 ASHP Technical Assistance Bulletin (Abridged)

RL 2.6: Aseptic technique and product preparation. All recommendations for risk level 1 sterile production preparation should be met.

A master work sheet should be developed for each batch of sterile products to be prepared. Once approved by the designated pharmacist, a verified duplicate (e.g., photocopy) of the master work sheet should be used as the preparation work sheet from which each batch is prepared and on which all documentation for that batch occurs. A separate preparation work sheet should be used for each batch prepared. The master work sheet should consist of the formula, components, compounding directions or procedures, a sample label, and evaluation and testing requirements. The preparation work sheet should be used to document the following:

1. Identity of all solutions and ingredients and their corresponding amounts, concentrations, or volumes;

2. Manufacturer lot number for each component;

3. Component manufacturer or suitable identifying number;

4. Container specifications (e.g., syringe, pump cassette);

5. Lot or control number assigned to batch;

6. Expiration date of batch-prepared products;

7. Date of preparation;

8. Identity (e.g., initials, codes, signatures) of personnel involved in preparation;

9. End-product evaluation and testing specifications;

10. Storage requirements;

11. Specific equipment used during aseptic preparation (e.g., a specific automated compounding device); and

12. Comparison of actual yield to anticipated yield, when appropriate.

A policy and procedure could be developed that allows separate documentation of batch formulas, compounding instructions, and records. However documentation is done, a procedure should exist for easy retrieval of all records pertaining to a particular batch. Each group of sterile batch-prepared products should bear a unique lot number. Under no circumstances should identical lot numbers be assigned to different products or different batches of the same product. Lot numbers may be alphabetic, numeric, or alphanumeric.

The process of combining multiple sterile ingredients into a single, sterile reservoir for subdivision into multiple units for dispensing may necessitate additional quality control procedures. It is recommended that calculations associated with this process be verified by a second pharmacist, when possible; this verification should be documented. Because this process often involves making multiple entries into the intermediate sterile reservoir, the likelihood of contamination may be greater than that associated with the preparation of other risk level 2 sterile products.

RL 2.7: Process validation. Each individual involved in the preparation of risk level 2 sterile products should successfully complete a validation process, as recommended for risk level 1. Process simulation procedures for compounding risk level 2 sterile products should be representative of all types of manipulations, products, and batch sizes that personnel preparing risk level 2 sterile products are likely to encounter.

DISCUSSION POINTS

Please read the preceding ASHP TAB 4.3–4.4 before you continue.

4.3 Aseptic Technique and Product Preparation

All of the recommendations for risk level 1 should be met. Risk level 2 quality assurance measures builds on risk level 1 (noted in **bold** print).

RL 2.6 Aseptic technique and product preparation

◊ all aseptic procedures should be performed at least 6 inches inside the laminar-airflow hood.

◊ do not overcrowd the critical work area.

◊ make sure the number of units is consistent with amount of work space in critical area.

◊ all ingredients should be stable, compatible and appropriate for product that is being prepared.

◊ do not use expired, inappropriately stored or defective products when preparing sterile products.

◊ when using automated compounding devices for preparation, verify data entered by pharmacist.

ADDITIONALLY...

◊ *a master worksheet should be prepared for each batch of sterile products to be prepared. A verified duplicate should be made as the preparation work sheet from which each batch is used.*

The following elements should be included on the preparation worksheet for risk level 2.

PREPARATION WORKSHEET

- identity of all solutions and ingredients and their corresponding amounts, concentrations, or volumes
- manufacturer lot number for each component
- component manufacturer or suitable identifying number
- container specifications
- lot or control number assigned to batch
- expiration date of batch-prepared products
- date of preparation
- identity of personnel involved in preparation
- end-product evaluation and testing specifications
- storage requirements
- specific equipment used during aseptic preparation
- comparison of actual yield to anticipated yield, when appropriate

---

Patient :
RX # : 700-4 Gentamicin 40MG/ML 2.75ML
Fill Date : 04/05/94
Next Fill : 04/09/94
Sched Ship : 04/05/94

Physician :
Entered by : TRF 03/11/94
Filled by : LPC 04/05/94
Approved by : TRF 04/05/94
CMPD Lot # :

Prepare: # Units : 10
Days Supply : 5
Admin Freq : Every 12 hours

Doses/Unit : 1
Total # Doses : 10

Compounding Instructions:
Stability: 14 days Refrig. Ref: _____

Expires on : 04/19/94

Prescription #: 700-4 Gentamicin 40MG/ML 2.75ML

ITEM	MFG	AMT/UNIT	XUNITS/FREQ	=	TOTAL
Gentamicin 40MG/ML	SoloPak	2.75ML	10		27.5ML
Sod Chloridesolno .9%	Baxter	50.00ML	10		500.0ML

INVENTORY PICK LIST

COMPONENTS	MFG	AMT/UNIT	VOL/UNIT	TOT VOL	CODE	PKG Size	Qty	Pick	Used	Lot #	Exp Date
Gentamicin 40MG/ML	SoloPak	110.00MG	2.75	27.5	181292913	2ML	14	14	14	1439	9/1/95
Sod Chloridesolno .9%	Baxter		50.0	500.0	140120046	50ML	10	10	10	6127	10/95

Rx: 700   04/05/94
Gentamicin Sulfate 110 MG
0.9% Sodium Chloride 50.0 MG

Infuse one bag over 10 minutes every 12 hours

Dr.
RFH: TRF   Doses: 10
Keep Refridgerated
Exp. 04/19/94

Prep Init: _____   Check Init: _____

4.4 Process Validation

Process simulation procedures for compounding risk level 2 sterile products should be representative of all types of manipulations, products, and batch sizes that personnel are likely to encounter.

RL 2.7: Process Validation

```
┌─────────────────────────────┐
│ Process medium as if it were a │
│ product                     │
└─────────────────────────────┘
              │
              ▼
┌─────────────────────────────┐
│ Incubate - then             │
│ evaluate                    │
└─────────────────────────────┘
              │
              ▼
┌─────────────────────────────┐
│ Was microbial               │
│ growth detected?            │
└─────────────────────────────┘
   If                      If
   yes                     no
   │                        │
   ▼                        ▼
┌──────────────────┐  ┌──────────────────┐
│ Process evaluated │  │ Adequate aseptic │
│ Correction made   │  │ technique used   │
│ Perform again     │  │                  │
└──────────────────┘  └──────────────────┘
```

TIPS

➤ Since most home care preparations fall in RL 2 or RL 3, the preparation worksheet is crucial to proper compounding and documentation. Many computer programs provide very complete worksheets (a.k.a. compounding sheets or mixing reports).

➤ When possible, a patient label on a worksheet greatly enhances documentation.

EXERCISES

1. List a minimum of 7 items which should be found on a preparation worksheet.

   _____

   _____

   _____

   _____

2. Examine your departmental procedure for process validation. Does it meet the recommendations for risk level 2? If not, describe what steps it may be lacking.

   _____

   _____

   _____

   _____

SELF-ASSESSMENT QUESTIONS

1. It is acceptable to use the same lot number for different batches of the same product.
   a. True
   b. False

2. If an automated compounding device is used in preparation of a product, this needs to be noted on the worksheet.
   a. True
   b. False

3. Process validation procedures for RL 2 should mimic all types of manipulations encountered in RL 2.
   a. True
   b. False

Please return to the videotape.

4.5 ASHP Technical Assistance Bulletin (Abridged)

RL 2.8: Expiration dating. All recommendations for risk level 1 should be met.

RL 2.9: Labeling. All recommendations for risk level 1 should be met.

RL 2.10: End-product evaluation. All recommendations for risk level 1 should be met. Additionally, the growth media fill procedure should be supplemented with a program of end-product sterility testing, according to a formal sampling plan. Written policies and procedures should specify measurements and methods of testing. Policies and procedures should include a statistically valid sampling plan and acceptance criteria for the sampling and testing. The criteria should be statistically adequate to reasonably ensure that the entire batch meets all specifications. Products not meeting all specifications should be rejected and discarded.

There should be a mechanism for recalling all products of a specific batch if end-product testing procedures yield unacceptable results. On completion of final testing, products should be stored in a manner that ensures their identity, strength, quality, and purity. Detailed information on end-product sterility testing is published elsewhere.

RL 2.11: Documentation. All recommendations for risk level 1 should be met. Additionally, documentation of end-product sampling and batch-preparation records should be maintained for an adequate period of time, according to organizational policies and procedures and state regulatory requirements. Documentation for sterile batch-prepared products should include the

1. Master work sheet;

2. Preparation work sheet; and

3. End-product evaluation and testing results.

DISCUSSION POINTS

Please read the preceding ASHP TAB 4.5 before you continue.

4.5 Expiration Dating, Labeling, End-product Evaluation, Documentation

All of the recommendations for risk level 1 should be met. Risk level 2 quality assurance measures builds on risk level 1 (noted in **bold** print).

RL 2.8: Expiration dating

◊ assigning an expiration date to a pharmacy-prepared sterile product should be done following an established procedure yet easy to implement and follow.

◊ evaluation of expiration dates should be done on a product by product basis and be based on currently available drug stability information and sterility considerations.

◊ when interpreting this information, consider all aspects of final sterile product such as *drug reservoir, drug concentration, storage conditions.*

◊ methods for establishing expiration dates should be documented

◊ appropriate in-house (or contract service) stability testing may be used to determine expiration dates

---

RL 2.9: Labeling

Remember to label sterile products with at least the following:
◊ patient name and identification (if patient-specific)
◊ control or lot number (if batch-prepared)
◊ all solution & ingredient names, amounts, strengths, and concentrations
◊ expiration date (and time when applicable)
◊ prescribed administration regimen including rate and route
◊ appropriate auxiliary labeling
◊ storage requirements
◊ identification of pharmacist
◊ device-specific instructions
◊ state or federal information

All recommendations should be met for risk level one. The value of end product evaluation is to verify that your process is sterile.

RL 2.10: End product evaluation

The end-product should be evaluated for:

◊ container leaks

◊ container integrity

◊ solution cloudiness

◊ particulates in the solution

◊ appropriate solution color

◊ solution volume when preparation is completed product dispensed

◊ verification that product was compounded accurately

ADDITIONALLY...

◊ *end-product sterility testing according to a formal sampling plan should supplement a growth media fill procedure.*

◊ *established mechanism for recalling all products of specific batch if end-product testing yields unacceptable results.*

Additional documentation should be included with those specified in recommendations for risk level one.

RL 2.11: Documentation

◊ training and competency evaluation of employees in sterile product procedures

◊ refrigerator and freezer temperatures

◊ certification of laminar-airflow hoods

◊ dispensing records for sterile products, in accordance with state regulatory requirements

ADDITIONALLY...

◊ *documentation of end-product sampling and batch-preparation record should be maintained for an adequate period of time.*

◊ *documentation for sterile batch-prepared products should include the master work sheet, preparation work sheet and end-product evaluation and testing results.*

SUMMARY

As you learned in section three, most of your pharmacy-prepared sterile products will fall within risk levels 1 or 2. The primary difference between risk level 1 and risk level 2 classification relates to administration and storage times. Because of this, changes in environmental monitoring policies, personnel training, facilities requirements and garb are among the more important differences from risk level 1 requirements.

TIPS

➤ Establish a manual with all standard expiration dates for compounded products used in your institution. Include references where applicable. Developing this will be a long, painstaking process, but it will be a valuable reference.

EXERCISES

1. List 3 aspects crucial to the interpretation of expiration dating of sterile products.

   _____

   _____

   _____

   _____

2. List 5 items on end-products that should be evaluated.

   _____

   _____

   _____

   _____

SELF-ASSESSMENT QUESTIONS

1. When interpreting drug stability information, which of the following is considered in making expiration dating decisions:
   a. drug reservoir
   b. drug concentration
   c. storage conditions
   d. all of the above

2. If a pharmacy-prepared sterile product is appropriately compounded and checked for accuracy by a pharmacist, but the identification of that pharmacist is not on the label, it is still acceptable to dispense that product.
   a. True
   b. False

3. A batch-prepared product should always possess its own control or lot number.
   a. True
   b. False

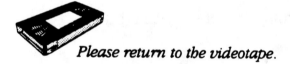

Please return to the videotape.

SECTION FIVE: QUALITY ASSURANCE FOR RISK LEVEL THREE

OVERVIEW

In the previous sections, you have learned the crucial steps to aseptic technique, risk level classification, and the quality assurance practices required for risk levels 1 and 2. In this section, the differences separating risk level 3 from levels 1 and 2 will be discussed.

OBJECTIVES

Upon completion of this section, you should be able to:

- Discuss why quality assurance activities are more demanding than risk level 1 or 2.

- In addition to risk levels 1 and 2, list at least 10 more policies and procedures specific to risk level 3 sterile products preparation.

- Identify personnel requirements for preparing products specific to risk level 3. Discuss 4 additional areas of knowledge a pharmacist should be proficient.

- Practice proper storage and handling requirements in accordance with manufacturer or USP requirements specific to risk level 3.

- Identify the higher standards for clean room requirements specific for risk level 3.

- Practice proper hygienic procedures when preparing sterile products to include use of gloves, gowns, masks and shoe covers.

- Describe risk levels 1 and 2 aseptic technique and product preparation to include higher standards for documentation, sterilization, and use of an integrity test for bacteria-retentive filter specific to risk level 3.

- Describe why process validation is important and how to conduct process simulation testing for risk level 3 sterile products.

- Employ a system that establishes proper assignment of substance expiration dates outlined in risk levels 1 and 2 to include laboratory testing of products for sterility, pyrogenicity, and chemical contents.

- Employ proper labeling guidelines for a prescription or medication order.

- Recognize product or container deficiency by an end-product evaluation for risk level 1 and 2.

- Conduct a systematic approach to essential documentation to include end-product sampling and batch-preparation records specific to risk level 3 sterile products.

5.1 ASHP Technical Assistance Bulletin (Abridged)

General comment on risk level 3. Risk level 3 addresses the preparation of products that pose the greatest potential risk to patients. The quality assurance activities described in this section are clearly more demanding—in terms of processes, facilities, and final product assessment—than for risk levels 1 and 2. Ideally, the activities described for risk level 3 would be used for all high-risk products. The activities may be viewed as most important in circumstances in which the medical need for such high-risk products is *routine*. In circumstances where the medical need for such a product is immediate (and there is not a suitable alternative) or when the preparation of such a product is rare, professional judgment must be applied as to the extent to which some activities (e.g., strict facility design, quarantine and final product testing before product dispensing) should be applied.

RL 3.1: Policies and procedures. There should be written policies and procedures related to every aspect of preparation of risk level 3 sterile products. These policies and procedures should be detailed enough to ensure that all products have the identity, strength, quality, and purity purported for the product. All policies and procedures should be reviewed and approved by the designated pharmacist. There should be a mechanism designed to ensure that policies and procedures are communicated, understood, and adhered to by personnel cleaning or working in the controlled area or support area. Policies and procedures should be reviewed at least annually by the designated pharmacist and department head. Written policies and procedures should define and identify the environmental monitoring activities necessary to ensure an adequate environment for risk level 3 sterile product preparation.

In addition to the policies and procedures required for risk levels 1 and 2, there should be written policies and procedures for the following:

1. Component handling and storage;

2. Any additional personnel qualifications commensurate with the preparation of risk level 3 sterile products;

3. Personnel responsibilities in the controlled area (e.g., cleaning, maintenance, access to controlled area);

4. Equipment use, maintenance, calibration, and testing;

5. Sterilization;

6. Master formula and master work sheet development and use;

7. End-product evaluation and testing;

8. Appropriate documentation for preparation of risk level 3 sterile products;

9. Use, control, and monitoring of environmentally controlled areas and calibration of monitoring equipment;

10. Validation of processes for preparing risk level 3 sterile products;

11. Quarantine of products and release from quarantine, if applicable;

12. A mechanism for recall of products from patients in the event that end-product testing procedures yield unacceptable results; and

13. Any other quality control procedures unique to the preparation of risk level 3 sterile products.

RL 3.2: Personnel education, training, and evaluation. Persons preparing sterile products at risk level 3 must have specific education, training, and experience to perform all functions required for the preparation of risk level 3 sterile products. However, final responsibility should lie with the pharmacist, who should be knowledgeable in the principles of good manufacturing practices and profi-

cient in quality assurance requirements, equipment used in the preparation of risk level 3 sterile products, and other aspects of sterile product preparation. The pharmacist should have sufficient education, training, experience, and demonstrated competency to ensure that all sterile products prepared from sterile or nonsterile components have the identity, strength, quality, and purity purported for the products. In addition to the body of knowledge required for risk levels 1 and 2, the pharmacist should possess sufficient knowledge in the following areas:

1. Aseptic processing;

2. Quality control and quality assurance as related to environmental, component, and end-product testing;

3. Sterilization techniques; and

4. Container, equipment, and closure system selection.

All pharmacy personnel involved in the cleaning and maintenance of the controlled area should be specially trained and thoroughly knowledgeable in the special requirements of Class 100 critical-area technology and design. There should be documented, ongoing training for all employees to enable retention of expertise.

DISCUSSION POINTS

Please read the preceding ASHP TAB 5.1 before you continue.

5.1 Policies and Procedures, Personnel Education, Training, and Evaluation

Risk level 3 recommendations are most important when preparation of high-risk products is *non-sterile* and *routine*. The quality assurance activities for risk level 3, addressing the preparation of products that pose the greatest potential risk to patients, build on the risk levels 1 and 2. In addition to the policies and procedures outlined in risk levels 1 and 2 there are additional items that are particular to risk 3 product preparation (noted in **bold** print).

RL 3.1: Policies and procedures

◊ personnel education and training requirements
◊ competency evaluation
◊ product acquisition
◊ storage and handling of products and supplies
◊ storage and delivery of final products
◊ use and maintenance of facilities and equipment
◊ appropriate garb and conduct for personnel working in controlled area
◊ process validation
◊ preparation technique
◊ labeling
◊ documentation
◊ quality control
◊ define and identify necessary environmental monitoring devices and techniques such as air velocity, temperature meters, and agar plates

ADDITIONALLY...

◊ *component handling and storage*
◊ *any additional personnel qualifications commensurate with the preparation of risk level 3 sterile products*
◊ *personnel responsibilities in the controlled area (e.g., cleaning, maintenance, access to controlled area)*
◊ *equipment use, maintenance, calibration, and testing*
◊ *sterilization*
◊ *master formula and master work sheet development and use*
◊ *end-product evaluation and testing*
◊ *appropriate documentation for preparation of risk level 3 sterile products*
◊ *use, control, and monitoring of environmentally controlled areas and calibration of monitoring equipment*
◊ *validation of processes for preparing risk level 3 sterile products*
◊ *quarantine of products and release from quarantine, if applicable*
◊ *a mechanism for recall of products from patients in the event that end-product testing procedures yield unacceptable results*
◊ *any other quality control procedures unique to the preparation of risk level 3 sterile products*

Please note that the final responsibility for handling any risk level 3 products ultimately is with the pharmacist. In addition to the knowledge areas required in risk levels 1 and 2 highlighted here, the pharmacist should be proficient in quality assurance requirements and equipment used in the preparation of risk level 3 sterile products.

RL 3.2: Personnel education, training and evaluation

◊ aseptic technique
◊ critical-area contamination factors
◊ environmental monitoring
◊ facilities, equipment, and supplies
◊ sterile product calculations and terminology
◊ sterile product compounding documentation
◊ quality assurance procedures
◊ aseptic preparation procedures
◊ proper gowning and gloving technique
◊ general conduct in the controlled area
◊ principles of "Current Good Manufacturing Practices"
◊ cleanroom design
◊ basic concepts of aseptic compounding
◊ critical-area contamination factors
◊ periodically assess all personnel preparing risk level 2 products through appropriate process simulation procedure.

ADDITIONALLY...
◊ *aseptic processing*
◊ *quality control and quality assurance as related to environmental, component, and end-product testing*
◊ *sterilization techniques*
◊ *container, equipment, and closure system selection*

TIPS

➤ Remember that risk level 3 guidelines are required when such product preparation is *routine*.

➤ Non-routine preparation of risk level 3 products may be performed in risk level 1 and 2 environments when, in a pharmacist's best judgement, it is considered necessary (e.g., an emergency medication).

EXERCISES

In order to complete these exercises, you should have the following materials available:

✳ your institution's policies and procedures manual

1. Review your policies and procedures manual to determine if quality assurance practices for risk level 3 product preparation are included.

2. Explain how the additional risk level 3 requirements for education and training are met by your department.

   _____

   _____

   _____

   _____

3. Explain your policies and procedures for recalling products that have failed end-product evaluation. Are they adequate for risk level 3 products?

   _____

   _____

   _____

   _____

SELF-ASSESSMENT QUESTIONS

1. In general, risk level 3 classification relates only to those products prepared on a non-routine basis, regardless of product ingredients or storage condition
    a. True
    b. False

2. End-product sterilization will always be required for risk level 3 products
    a. True
    b. False

3. A pharmacist preparing risk level 3 products should possess sufficient knowledge in the following areas: sterilization techniques; quality control and quality assurance as related to environmental, component, and end-product testing; and container, equipment, and closure system selection.

    a. True
    b. False

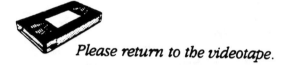

Please return to the videotape.

5.2 ASHP Technical Assistance Bulletin (Abridged)

RL 3.3: Storage and handling. In addition to recommendations for risk levels 1 and 2, risk level 3 policies and procedures for storage and handling should include the procurement, identification, storage, handling, testing, and recall of components and finished products.

Components and finished products ready to undergo end-product testing should be stored in a manner that prevents their use before release by a pharmacist, minimizes the risk of contamination, and enables identification. There should be identifiable storage areas that can be used to quarantine products, if necessary, before they are released.

RL 3.4: Facilities and equipment. Preparation of risk level 3 sterile products should occur in a Class 100 horizontal- or vertical-laminar-airflow hood that is properly situated in a controlled area that meets Class 10,000 conditions for acceptable airborne particle levels *or* in a properly maintained and monitored Class 100 cleanroom (without the hood). The controlled area should have a positive pressure differential relative to adjacent, less clean areas of at least 0.05 inch of water. Solutions that are to be terminally sterilized may be prepared in a Class 100 laminar-airflow hood located inside a controlled area that meets Class 100,000 conditions.

To allow proper cleaning and disinfection, walls, floors, and ceilings in the controlled area should be nonporous. To help reduce the number of particles in the controlled area, an adjacent support area (e.g., anteroom) should be provided.

During the preparation of risk level 3 sterile products, access to the controlled area or cleanroom should be limited to those individuals who are required to be in the area and are properly attired. The environment of the main access areas directly adjacent to the controlled area (e.g., anteroom) should meet at least Federal Standard 209E Class 100,000 requirements. To help maintain a Class 100 critical-area environment during compounding, the adjacent support area (e.g., anteroom) should be separated from the controlled area by a barrier (e.g., plastic curtain, partition, wall). Written policies and procedures for monitoring the environment of the controlled area and adjacent areas should be developed.

No sterile products should be prepared in the controlled area if it fails to meet established criteria specified in the policies and procedures. A calibrated particle counter capable of measuring air particles 0.5 mm and larger should be used to monitor airborne particulate matter. Before product preparation begins, the positive-pressure air status should meet or exceed the requirements. Air samples should be taken at several places in the controlled area with the appropriate environmental monitoring devices (e.g., nutrient agar plates). Surfaces on which work actually occurs, including laminar-airflow hood surfaces and tabletops, should be monitored using surface contact plates, the swab-rinse technique, or other appropriate methods.

Test results should be reviewed and criteria should be pre-established to determine the point at which the preparation of risk level 3 sterile products will be disallowed until corrective measures are taken. When the environment does not meet the criteria specified in the policies and procedures, sterile product processing should immediately cease and corrective action should be taken. In the event that this occurs, written policies and procedures should delineate alternative methods of sterile product preparation to enable timely fulfillment of prescription orders.

Equipment should be adequate to prevent microbiological contamination. Methods should be established for the cleaning, preparation, sterilization, calibration, and documented use of all equipment.

Critical-area work surfaces should be disinfected with an appropriate agent before the preparation of each product. Floors in the controlled area should be disinfected at least daily. Exterior hood surfaces and other hard surfaces in the controlled area, such as shelves, tables, and stools, should be disinfected weekly and after any unanticipated event that could increase the risk of contamination. Walls and ceilings in the controlled area or cleanroom should be disinfected at least weekly.

Large pieces of equipment, such as tanks, carts, and tables, used in the controlled area or cleanroom should be made of a material that can be easily cleaned and disinfected; stainless steel is recommended. Equipment that does not come in direct contact with the finished product should be properly cleaned, rinsed, and disinfected before being placed in the controlled area. All nonsterile equipment that will come in contact with the sterilized final product should be properly sterilized before introduction into the controlled area; this precaution includes such items as tubing, filters, containers, and other processing equipment. The sterilization process should be monitored and documented.

RL 3.5: Garb. All recommendations for risk levels 1 and 2 should be met. Additionally, cleanroom garb should be worn inside the controlled area at all times during the preparation of risk level 3 sterile products. Attire should consist of a low-shedding coverall, head cover, face mask, and shoe covers. These garments may be either disposable or reusable. Head and facial hair should be covered. Before donning these garments over street clothes, personnel should thoroughly wash their hands and arms up to the elbows with a suitable antimicrobial skin cleanser. Sterile disposable gloves should be worn and rinsed frequently with an appropriate agent (e.g., 70% isopropyl alcohol) during processing. The gloves should be changed if the integrity is compromised. If persons leave the controlled area *or support area* during processing, they should regown with clean garments before re-entering.

DISCUSSION POINTS

Please read the preceding ASHP TAB 5.2 before you continue.

5.2 Storage and Handling, Facilities and Equipment, Garb

In addition to recommendations for risk levels 1 and 2, the following are necessary for the handling of risk level 3 products (noted in **bold** print):

RL 3.3: Storage and handling

◊ solutions, drugs, supplies, and equipment used to prepare or administer sterile products should be stored in accordance with manufacturer or USP requirements.

◊ refrigerator and freezer temperatures should be monitored and documented daily to meet compendial storage requirements.

◊ storage areas were ingredients are stored should be monitored to ensure temperature, light, moisture, and ventilation remain within manufacturer and compendial requirements.

◊ drugs and supplies should be stored on shelving areas above floor.

◊ remove all products that have exceeded their expiration dates

◊ inspect each drug, ingredient and container for damage, defects and expiration date.

◊ keep unnecessary personnel traffic in controlled area to minimum

◊ packaging of materials and items generating unacceptable amounts of particles should not be permitted in controlled area.

◊ keep controlled area sanitized by daily disposals of used syringes, containers, and needles.

◊ initiate system for tracking and retrieving affected products from patients to whom they were dispensed.

ADDITIONALLY...

◊ ***procure, identify, store, handle, test, and recall components and finished products.***

RL 3.4: Facilities and equipment

◊ controlled area should have limited access and be separated from other pharmacy operations.

◊ controlled area should be clean, well lighted, and of sufficient size to support sterile compounding activities.

◊ clean and disinfect controlled areas at regular intervals including refrigerators, freezers and shelves where products are stored.

◊ a sink should be located nearby for hand washing.

◊ prepare all cytotoxic and other hazardous products in a Class II biological-safety cabinet or vertical hood environment.

◊ the exterior surfaces of the laminar-airflow hood should be cleaned periodically with a mild detergent or suitable disinfectant.

◊ cleaning materials should be made of materials that generate a low amount of particles.

◊ create an adjacent support area of high cleanliness and separate with barrier.

ADDITIONALLY...

◊ *prepare products in class 100 horizontal-or vertical-laminar-airflow hood situated in controlled area meeting Class 10,000 conditions for acceptable airborne particle levels or in Class 100 cleanroom (without hood).*

◊ *controlled area should have positive pressure differential relative to adjacent, less clean areas of at least 0.05 inch of water.*

◊ *solutions terminally sterilized may be prepared in Class 100 laminar-airflow hood located inside a controlled area meeting Class 100,000 conditions.*

◊ *walls, floors, and ceilings in controlled area should be nonporous.*

◊ *provide adjacent support area to reduce number of particles in controlled area.*

◊ *limit access to controlled area or cleanroom.*

◊ *no sterile products should be prepared in controlled area if fail to meet established criteria.*

◊ *air samples should be taken at several places in controlled areas with appropriate environmental monitoring devices.*

◊ *review and refine policies and procedures for testing.*

◊ *all equipment should be adequate to prevent microbiological contamination.*

◊ *critical-area work surfaces should be disinfected with appropriate agent before preparation of each product.*

◊ *large pieces of equipment used in controlled area or cleanroom should be made of easily cleaned material.*

> ### RL 3.5: Garb
> ◊ personnel should wear clean clothing covers that generate low amounts of particles in the controlled area.
> ◊ cover your head and facial hair and wear a mask during all aseptic preparation procedures.
> ◊ scrub to the elbow with an appropriate anti microbial skin cleanser.
> ◊ gloves, gowns and masks and shoe covers are recommended.
>
> ***ADDITIONALLY...***
>
> ◊ ***cleanroom garb should be worn inside cleanroom at all times during product preparation.***

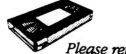

Please return to the videotape.

TIPS

➤ Be sure that more than one pharmacist is familiar with the procedures for obtaining necessary non-sterile ingredients used in preparing risk level 3 products. If this is generally the responsibility of one person, have a written process detailing how these ingredients can be obtained in an emergency situation.

➤ If your department plans to remodel your controlled room, be aware of the garb your employees will be wearing. Gowns can be restrictive; be sure to design the work area to allow plenty of free movement.

EXERCISES

1. Review your department's recall policy and procedures. Is it in keeping with risk level 3 requirements? If not, identify those steps that need to be revised.

   _____

   _____

   _____

2. Take air samples of your controlled room to determine if it meets the conditions outlined in risk level 3 recommendations.

SELF-ASSESSMENT QUESTIONS

1. Products that fall under risk level 3 should be prepared in a Class 100 laminar-airflow hood located in a controlled area that meets Class 10,000 conditions.

   a. True

   b. False

2. All risk level 3 products must be quarantined until end-product testing is performed.

   a. True

   b. False

3. When preparing risk level 3 products, reusable garb should not be worn.

   a. True

   b. False

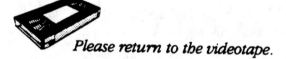

Please return to the videotape.

5.3 ASHP Technical Assistance Bulletin (Abridged)

RL 3.6: Aseptic technique and product preparation. All recommendations for risk levels 1 and 2 should be met. Methods should ensure that components and containers remain free from contamination and are easily identified as to the product, lot number, and expiration date. If components are not finished sterile pharmaceuticals obtained from licensed manufacturers, pharmacists should ensure that these components meet USP standards. Products prepared from nonsterile ingredients should be tested to ensure that they do not exceed specified endotoxin limits. As each new lot of components and containers is received, the components should be quarantined until properly identified, tested, or verified by a pharmacist.

The methods for preparing sterile products and using process controls should be designed to ensure that finished products have the identity, strength, quality, and purity they are intended to have. Any deviations from established methods should be documented and appropriately justified.

A master work sheet should be developed for the preparation of each risk level 3 sterile product. Once approved by the pharmacist, a verified duplicate of the master work sheet should be used as the controlling document from which each sterile end product or batch of prepared products is compounded and on which all documentation for that product or batch occurs. The master work sheet should document all the requirements for risk level 2 plus the following:

1. Comparison of actual with anticipated yield;

2. Sterilization method(s); and

3. Quarantine specifications.

The preparation work sheet should serve as the batch record for each time a risk level 3 sterile product is prepared. Each batch of pharmacy-prepared sterile products should bear a unique lot number, as described in risk level 2.

There should be documentation on the preparation work sheet of all additions of individual components plus the signatures or initials of those individuals involved with the measuring or weighing and addition of these components.

The selection of the final packaging system (including container and closure) for the sterile product is crucial to maintaining product integrity. To the extent possible, presterilized containers obtained from licensed manufacturers should be used. If an aseptic filling operation is used, the container should be sterile at the time of the filling operation. If nonsterile containers are used, methods for sterilizing these containers should be established. Final containers selected should be capable of maintaining product integrity (i.e., identity, strength, quality, and purity) throughout the shelf life of the product.

For products requiring sterilization, selection of an appropriate method of sterilization is of prime importance. Methods of product sterilization include sterile filtration, autoclaving, dry heat sterilization, chemical sterilization, and irradiation. Selection of the sterilization technique should be based on the properties of the product being processed. The pharmacist must ensure that the sterilization method used is appropriate for the product components and does not alter the pharmaceutical properties of the final product. A method of sterilization often used by pharmacists is sterile filtration. In sterile filtration, the product should be filtered into presterilized containers un-

der aseptic conditions. Sterilizing filters of 0.22 mm or smaller porosity should be used in this process. Colloidal or viscous products may require use of a 0.45-mm filter; however, extreme caution should be exercised in these circumstances, and more stringent end-product sterility testing is essential.

To ensure that a bacteria-retentive filter did not rupture during filtration of a product, an integrity test should be performed on all filters immediately after filtration. This test may be accomplished by performing a bubble point test, in which pressurized gas is applied to the upstream side of the filter with the downstream outlet immersed in water and the pressure at which a steady stream of bubbles begins to appear is noted. The observed pressure is then compared with the manufacturer's specification for the filter. To compare the used filter with the manufacturer's specifications, which would be based on the filtration of water through the filter, it is necessary to first rinse the filter with sterile water for injection. An observed value lower than the manufacturer's specification indicates that the filter was defective or ruptured during the sterilization process. Methods should be established for handling, testing, and resterilizing any product processed with a filter that fails the integrity test.

RL 3.7: Process validation. In addition to risk level 1 and 2 recommendations, written policies and procedures should be established to validate all processes involved in the preparation of risk level 3 sterile products (including all procedures, equipment, and techniques) from sterile or nonsterile components. In addition to evaluating personnel technique, process validation provides a mechanism for determining whether a particular process will, when performed by qualified personnel, consistently produce the intended results.

RL 3.8: Expiration dating. In addition to risk level 2 recommendations, there should be reliable methods for establishing all expiration dates including laboratory testing of products for sterility, pyrogenicity, and chemical content, when necessary. These tests should be conducted in a manner based on appropriate statistical criteria, and the results documented.

RL 3.9: Labeling. All recommendations for risk levels 1 and 2 should be met.

RL 3.10: End-product evaluation. For each preparation of a sterile product or a batch of sterile products, there should be appropriate laboratory determination of conformity with established written specifications and policies. Any reprocessed material should undergo complete final product testing. It is advisable to quarantine sterile products compounded from nonsterile components, pending the results of end-product testing. If products

prepared from nonsterile components must be dispensed before satisfactory completion of end-product testing, there must be a procedure to allow for immediate recall of the products from patients to whom they were dispensed.

RL 3.11: Documentation. In addition to the recommendations for risk levels 1 and 2, documentation for risk level 3 sterile products should include

1. Preparation work sheet;

2. Sterilization records of final products (if applicable);

3. Quarantine records (if applicable); and

4. End-product evaluation and testing results.

*Unless otherwise stated in this document, the term "sterile products" refers to sterile drug or nutritional substances that are prepared (e.g., compounded or repackaged) by pharmacy personnel.

DISCUSSION POINTS

Please read the preceding ASHP TAB 5.3 before you continue.

5.3 Aseptic Technique and Product Preparation, Process Validation, Expiration Dating, Labeling, End-Product Evaluation, Documentation

The following quality assurance recommendations build on risk levels 1 and 2. It is important to remember that all recommendations for risk level 1 and 2 must still be met. In most cases, the level of preparation, validation, and documentation for risk level 3 are much more intensive.

The following summary builds on risk levels 1 and 2 (noted in **bold**).

RL 3.6: Aseptic technique and product preparation

◊ all aseptic procedures should be performed at least 6 inches inside the laminar-airflow hood.

◊ do not overcrowd the critical work area.

◊ make sure the number of units is consistent with amount of work space in critical area.

◊ all ingredients should be stable, compatible and appropriate for product that is being prepared.

◊ do not use expired, inappropriately stored or defective products when preparing sterile products.

◊ when using automated compounding devices for preparation, verify data entered by pharmacist.

◊ a master worksheet should be prepared for each batch of sterile products to be prepared. A verified duplicate should be made as the preparation work sheet from which each batch is used.

ADDITIONALLY...

◊ *a master work sheet should document comparison of actual with anticipated yield, sterilization method, quarantine specifications.*

◊ *products prepared from non-sterile ingredients should be tested to ensure specified endotoxin limits not exceeded.*

◊ *select sterilization method based on properties of product being processed.*

As stated in RL 3.7 of the ASHP TAB, the important difference for **process validation** is the establishment of validation procedures for all processes in the preparation of risk level 3 products; **not** just the aseptic technique process. This, for example, would include validation of equipment used (e.g., balances), other techniques such as proper gowning, or procedures such as hand washing. While these practices are just as important for the preparation of all sterile products, they are critical for risk level 3.

RL 3.8: Expiration dating

◊ assigning an expiration date to a pharmacy-prepared sterile product should be done following an established procedure yet easy to implement and follow.

◊ evaluation of expiration dates should be done on a product by product basis and be based on currently available drug stability information and sterility considerations.

◊ when interpreting this information, consider all aspects of final sterile product such as *drug reservoir, drug concentration, storage conditions.*

◊ methods for establishing expiration dates should be documented

◊ appropriate in-house (or contract service) stability testing may be used to determine expiration dates

ADDITIONALLY...

◊ *establish reliable methods for expiration dates including laboratory testing of products for sterility, pyrogenicity, and chemical content.*

RL 3.9: Labeling

◊ patient name and identification (if patient-specific)

◊ control or lot number (if batch-prepared)

◊ all solution & ingredient names, amounts, strengths, and concentrations

◊ expiration date (and time when applicable)

◊ prescribed administration regimen including rate and route

◊ appropriate auxiliary labeling

◊ storage requirements

◊ identification of pharmacist

◊ device-specific instructions

◊ state or federal information

The end-product should be evaluated for:

RL 3.10: End-product evaluation

◊ container leaks

◊ container integrity

◊ solution cloudiness

◊ particulates in the solution

◊ appropriate solution color

◊ solution volume when preparation is completed product dispensed

◊ verification that product was compounded accurately

◊ end-product sterility testing according to a formal sampling plan should supplement a growth media fill procedure.

◊ established mechanism for recalling all products of specific batch if end-product testing yields unacceptable results.

ADDITIONALLY...

◊ ***establish written specifications and policies for appropriate laboratory determination of conformity for each preparation of sterile product or batch of sterile products.***

RL 3.11: Documentation

◊ training and competency evaluation of employees in sterile product procedures

◊ refrigerator and freezer temperatures

◊ certification of laminar-airflow hoods

◊ dispensing records for sterile products, in accordance with state regulatory requirements

◊ documentation of end-product sampling and batch-preparation record should be maintained for an adequate period of time.

◊ documentation for sterile batch-prepared products should include the master work sheet, preparation work sheet and end-product evaluation and testing results.

ADDITIONALLY...

◊ ***preparation work sheet***

◊ ***sterilization records of final products***

◊ ***quarantine records***

◊ ***end-product evaluation and testing results***

SUMMARY

The ASHP TAB classifies sterile product preparation into three risk level classifications. In most instances, product preparation will fall within risk levels 1 and 2. However, for some products, risk level 3 quality assurance practices will be required. These guidelines are much more stringent, and require a higher level of training, validation, and documentation. The final determination of placing a product into risk level 3 may be dependent on the need for the product and situation in which it is being used. It falls upon the pharmacist to use his or her best judgement to take final responsibility for risk level classification.

TIPS

➤ If your department uses filtration as a means of end-product filtration, be sure to demonstrate to all new employees, the amount of time this procedure can take. It is important that new employees understand how slow this process can be, so they do not try to force the fluid through the filter and risk having the filter being forced off the syringe.

➤ Make sure that all pharmacy employees, not only those involved in the preparation of sterile products, understand the concept of a quarantined area. Make it clear that other items (e.g., food) should not be stored in the quarantine area.

EXERCISES

1. Prepare a master worksheet and preparation worksheet for a risk level 3 product.

2. Randomly select a recently prepared risk level 3 product and follow your department procedures to recall this product. If this could not easily be accomplished, identify the steps in your policy that must be corrected.

SELF-ASSESSMENT QUESTIONS

1. A master worksheet should document comparison of actual with anticipated yield, filtration method, and quarantine specifications.
   a. True
   b. False

2. The important difference between risk level 3 and risk level 2 process validation is the establishment of validation procedures for all processes in the preparation of risk level 3 products; not just aseptic processing.
   a. True
   b. False

3. Documentation for risk level 3 must include copies of all appropriate manufacturer safety data sheets (MSDS).
   a. True
   b. False

Appendix 1

ASHP REPORTS

ASHP technical assistance bulletin on quality assurance for pharmacy-prepared sterile products

Am J Hosp Pharm. 1993; 50:2386-98

Pharmacists are responsible for the correct preparation of sterile products.a Patient morbidity and mortality have resulted from incorrectly prepared or contaminated pharmacy-prepared products.1-5 These ASHP recommendations are intended to help pharmacists ensure that pharmacy-prepared sterile products are of high quality.

The National Coordinating Committee on Large Volume Parenterals (NCCLVP), which ceased to exist in the 1980s, published a series of recommendations in the 1970s and early 1980s,[6-12] including an article on quality assurance (QA) for centralized intravenous admixture services in hospitals.[7] The NCCLVP recommendations, however, are somewhat dated and do not cover the variety of settings in which pharmacists practice today nor the many types of sterile preparations pharmacists compound in current practice settings.

The Joint Commission on Accreditation of Healthcare Organizations (JCAHO) publishes only general standards relating to space, equipment and supplies, and record keeping for the preparation of sterile products in hospitals.[13] The 1993 JCAHO home care standards provide somewhat more detailed, nationally recognized pharmaceutical standards for home care organizations.[14] These standards, however, also lack sufficient detail to provide pharmacists with adequate information on quality assurance activities.

The Food and Drug Administration (FDA) publishes regulations on Current Good Manufacturing Practices [15,16] that apply to sterile products made by pharmaceutical manufacturers for shipment in interstate commerce. The FDA has also published a draft guideline on the manufacture of sterile drug products by aseptic processing.[17] Both of these documents apply to the manufacture of sterile products by licensed pharmaceutical manufacturers. The Centers for Disease Control and Prevention (CDC) has published guidelines for hand washing, prevention of intravascular infections,[18] and hospital environmental control.[19] The United States Pharmacopeial Convention, Inc., (USPC) establishes drug standards for packaging and storage, labeling, identification, pH, particulate matter, heavy metals, assay, and other requirements[16]; as of this writing, there is an effort under way at USPC to develop an informational chapter on compounding sterile products intended for home use.[20]

Although the aforementioned guidelines provide assistance to pharmacists, each has certain limitations (e.g., outdated, limited scope). None of these guidelines addresses sterile product storage and administration with newer types of equipment (e.g., portable infusion devices,[21,22] indwelling medication reservoirs) or the use of automated sterile-product compounding devices.[23]

This document was developed to help pharmacists establish quality assurance procedures for the preparation of sterile products. The recommendations in this Technical Assistance Bulletin are applicable to pharmacy services in various practice settings including but not limited to hospitals, community pharmacies, nursing homes, and home health care organizations. ASHP has published a practice standard on handling cytotoxic and hazardous drugs[24]; when preparing sterile preparations involving cytotoxic or hazardous drugs, pharmacists should consider the advice in that document.

The ASHP Technical Assistance Bulletin on Quality Assurance for Pharmacy-Prepared Sterile Products *does not* apply to the *manufacture* of sterile pharmaceuticals, as defined in state and federal laws and regulations, *nor* does it apply to the preparation of medications by pharmacists, nurses, or physicians in emergency situations for *immediate* administration to patients. Not all recommendations may be applicable to the preparation of pharmaceuticals.

These recommendations are referenced with supporting

Approved by the ASHP Board of Directors, September 24, 1993. Developed by the ASHP Council on Professional Affairs.

The assistance of the following individuals is acknowledged: . Clyde Buchanan, M.S.; Philip J. Schneider, M.S., FASHP; Howard Switzky; Lawrence A. Trissel, FASHP; and Larry Pelham, M.S.

scientific data when such data exist. In the absence of published supporting data, recommendations are based on expert opinion or generally accepted pharmacy procedures. Pharmacists are urged to use professional judgment in interpreting these recommendations and applying them in practice. It is recognized that, in certain emergency situations, a pharmacist may be requested to compound products under conditions that do not meet the recommendations. In such situations, it is incumbent upon the pharmacist to employ professional judgment in weighing the potential patient risks and benefits associated with the compounding procedure in question.

Objectives. The objectives of these recommendations are to provide

1. Information to pharmacists on quality assurance and quality control activities that may be applied to the preparation of sterile products in pharmacies; and
2. A scheme to match quality assurance and quality control activities with the potential risks to patients posed by various types of products.

Multidisciplinary input. Pharmacists are urged to participate in the quality improvement, risk management, and infection control programs of their organizations. In so doing, pharmacists should report findings about quality assurance in sterile preparations to the appropriate staff members or committees (e.g., risk management, infection control practitioners) when procedures that may lead to patient harm are known or suspected to be in use. Pharmacists should also cooperate with managers of quality improvement, risk management, and infection control to develop optimal sterile product procedures.

Definitions. Definitions of selected terms, as used for the purposes of this document, are located in the appendix. For brevity in this document, the term *quality assurance* will be used to refer to both quality assurance and quality control (as defined in the appendix), as befits the circumstances.

Risk level classification

In this document, sterile products are grouped into three levels of risk to the patient, increasing from least (level 1) to greatest (level 3) potential risk and having different associated quality assurance recommendations for product integrity and patient safety. This classification system should assist pharmacists in selecting which sterile product preparation procedures to use. Compounded sterile products in risk levels 2 and 3 should meet or exceed all of the quality assurance recommendations for risk level 1. When circumstances make risk level assignment unclear, recommendations for the higher risk level should prevail. Pharmacists must exercise their own professional judgment in deciding which risk level applies to a specific compounded sterile product or situation. Consideration should be given to factors that increase potential risk to the patient, such as multiple system breaks, compounding complexities, high-risk administration sites, immunocompromised status of the patient, use of nonsterile components, microbial growth potential of the finished sterile

drug product, storage conditions, and circumstances such as time between compounding and initiation of administration. The following risk assignments, based on the expertise of knowledgeable practitioners, represent one logical arrangement in which pharmacists may evaluate risk. Pharmacists may construct alternative arrangements that could be supported on the basis of scientific information and professional judgment.

Risk level 1. Risk level 1 applies to compounded sterile products that exhibit characteristics 1, 2, *and* 3 stated below. All risk level 1 products should be prepared with sterile equipment (e.g., syringes, vials), sterile ingredients and solutions, and sterile contact surfaces for the final product. Of the three risk levels, risk level 1 necessitates the least amount of quality assurance. Risk level 1 includes the following:

1. Products
   A. Stored at room temperature (see the appendix for temperature definitions) and completely administered within 28 hours from preparation; or
   B. Stored under refrigeration for 7 days or less before complete administration to a patient over a period not to exceed 24 hours (Table 1); or
   C. Frozen for 30 days or less before complete administration to a patient over a period not to exceed 24 hours.
2. Unpreserved sterile products prepared for administration to one patient, or batch-prepared products containing suitable preservatives prepared for administration to more than one patient.
3. Products prepared by closed-system aseptic transfer of sterile, nonpyrogenic, finished pharmaceuticals obtained from licensed manufacturers into sterile final containers (e.g., syringe, minibag, portable infusion-device cassette) obtained from licensed manufacturers.

Risk level 2. Risk level 2 sterile products exhibit characteristic 1, 2, *or* 3 stated below. All risk level 2 products should be prepared with sterile equipment, sterile ingredients and solutions, and sterile contact surfaces for the final product and by using closed-system transfer methods. Risk level 2 includes the following:

1. Products stored beyond 7 days under refrigeration, or stored beyond 30 days frozen, or administered beyond 28 hours after preparation and storage at room temperature (Table 1).
2. Batch-prepared products without preservatives that are intended for use by more than one patient. (Note: Batch-prepared products without preservatives that will be administered to multiple patients carry a greater risk to the patients than products prepared for a single patient because of the potential effect of product contamination on the health and well-being of a larger patient group.)
3. Products compounded by combining multiple sterile ingredients, obtained from licensed manufacturers, in a sterile reservoir, obtained from a licensed manufacturer, by using closed-system aseptic transfer before subdivision into multiple units to be dispensed to patients.

Risk level 3. Risk level 3 products exhibit either charac-

Table 1.

Assignment of Products to Risk Level 1 or 2 according to Time and Temperature before Completion of Administration

| Risk Level | Room Temperature (15 to 30 °C) | Days of Storage | |
		Refrigerator (2 to 8 °C)	Freezer (−20 to −10 °C)
1	Completely administered within 28 hr	≤7	≤30
2	Storage and administration exceeds 28 hr	>7	>30

teristic 1 *or* 2:

1. Products compounded from nonsterile ingredients or compounded with nonsterile components, containers, or equipment.
2. Products prepared by combining multiple ingredients—sterile or nonsterile—by using an open-system transfer or open reservoir before terminal sterilization or subdivision into multiple units to be dispensed.

Quality assurance for risk level 1

RL 1.1: Policies and procedures. Up-to-date policies and procedures for compounding sterile products should be written and available to all personnel involved in these activities. Policies and procedures should be reviewed at least annually by the designated pharmacist and department head and updated, as necessary, to reflect current standards of practice and quality. Additions, revisions, and deletions should be communicated to all personnel involved in sterile compounding and related activities. These policies and procedures should address personnel education and training requirements, competency evaluation, product acquisition, storage and handling of products and supplies, storage and delivery of final products, use and maintenance of facilities and equipment, appropriate garb and conduct for personnel working in the controlled area, process validation, preparation technique, labeling, documentation, and quality control.[9] Further, written policies and procedures should address personnel access and movement of materials into and near the controlled area. Policies and procedures for monitoring environmental conditions in the controlled area should take into consideration the amount of exposure of the product to the environment during compounding. Before compounding sterile products, all personnel involved should read the policies and procedures and sign to verify their understanding.

RL 1.2: Personnel education, training, and evaluation. Pharmacy personnel preparing or dispensing sterile products should receive suitable didactic and experiential training and competency evaluation through demonstration, testing (written or practical), or both. Some aspects that should be included in training programs include aseptic technique; critical-area contamination factors; environmental monitoring; facilities, equipment, and supplies; sterile

product calculations and terminology; sterile product compounding documentation; quality assurance procedures; aseptic preparation procedures; proper gowning and gloving technique; and general conduct in the controlled area. In addition to knowledge of chemical, pharmaceutical, and clinical properties of drugs, pharmacists should also be knowledgeable about the principles of Current Good Manufacturing Practices.[15,16] Videotapes[25] and additional information on the essential components of a training, orientation, and evaluation program are described elsewhere.[7,12,26,27] All pharmacy personnel involved in cleaning and maintenance of the controlled area should be knowledgeable about cleanroom design (if applicable), the basic concepts of aseptic compounding, and critical-area contamination factors. Nonpharmacy personnel (e.g., housekeeping staff) involved in the cleaning or maintenance of the controlled area should receive adequate training on applicable procedures.

The aseptic technique of each person preparing sterile products should be observed and evaluated as satisfactory during orientation and training and at least on an annual basis thereafter. In addition to observation, methods of evaluating the knowledge of personnel include written or practical tests and process validation.

RL 1.3: Storage and handling. Solutions, drugs, supplies, and equipment used to prepare or administer sterile products should be stored in accordance with manufacturer or USP requirements. Temperatures in refrigerators and freezers used to store ingredients and finished sterile preparations should be monitored and documented daily to ensure that compendial storage requirements are met. Warehouse and other pharmacy storage areas where ingredients are stored should be monitored to ensure that temperature, light, moisture, and ventilation remain within manufacturer and compendial requirements. To permit adequate floor cleaning, drugs and supplies should be stored on shelving areas above the floor. Products that have exceeded their expiration dates should be removed from active storage areas. Before use, each drug, ingredient, and container should be visually inspected for damage, defects, and expiration date.

Unnecessary personnel traffic in the controlled area should be minimized. Particle-generating activities, such as removal of intravenous solutions, drugs, and supplies from cardboard boxes, should not be performed in the controlled area. Products and supplies used in preparing sterile products should be removed from shipping containers outside the controlled area before aseptic processing is begun. Packaging materials and items generating unacceptable amounts of particles (e.g., cardboard boxes, paper towels, reference books) should not be permitted in the controlled area or critical area. The removal of immediate packaging designed to retain the sterility or stability of a product (e.g., syringe packaging, light-resistant pouches) is an exception; obviously, this type of packaging should not be removed outside the controlled area. Disposal of packaging materials, used syringes, containers, and needles should be performed at least daily, and more often if needed, to enhance sanitation and avoid accumulation in the controlled area.

In the event of a product recall, there should be a mechanism for tracking and retrieving affected products from specific patients to whom the products were dispensed.

RL 1.4: Facilities and equipment. The controlled area should be a limited-access area sufficiently separated from other pharmacy operations to minimize the potential for contamination that could result from the unnecessary flow of materials and personnel into and out of the area. Computer entry, order processing, label generation, and record keeping should be performed outside the critical area. The controlled area should be clean, well lighted, and of sufficient size to support sterile compounding activities. For hand washing, a sink with hot and cold running water should be in close proximity. Refrigeration, freezing, ventilation, and room temperature control capabilities appropriate for storage of ingredients, supplies, and pharmacy-prepared sterile products in accordance with manufacturer, USP, and state or federal requirements should exist. The controlled area should be cleaned and disinfected at regular intervals with appropriate agents, according to written policies and procedures. Disinfectants should be alternated periodically to prevent the development of resistant microorganisms. The floors of the controlled area should be nonporous and washable to enable regular disinfection. Active work surfaces in the controlled area (e.g., carts, compounding devices, counter surfaces) should be disinfected, in accordance with written procedures. Refrigerators, freezers, shelves, and other areas where pharmacy-prepared sterile products are stored should be kept clean.

Sterile products should be prepared in a Class 100 environment.[28] Such an environment exists inside a certified horizontal- or vertical-laminar-airflow hood. Facilities that meet the recommendations for risk level 3 preparation would be suitable for risk level 1 and 2 compounding. Cytotoxic and other hazardous products should be prepared in a Class II biological-safety cabinet.[24] Laminar-airflow hoods are designed to be operated continuously. If a laminar-airflow hood is turned off between aseptic processing, it should be operated long enough to allow complete purging of room air from the critical area (e.g., 15–30 minutes), then disinfected before use. The critical-area work surface and all accessible interior surfaces of the hood should be disinfected with an appropriate agent before work begins and periodically thereafter, in accordance with written policies and procedures. The exterior surfaces of the laminar-airflow hood should be cleaned periodically with a mild detergent or suitable disinfectant; 70% isopropyl alcohol may damage the hood's clear plastic surfaces. The laminar-airflow hood should be certified by a qualified contractor at least every six months or when it is relocated to ensure operational efficiency and integrity.[29] Prefilters in the laminar-airflow hood should be changed

periodically, in accordance with written policies and procedures.

A method should be established to calibrate and verify the accuracy of automated compounding devices used in aseptic processing.

RL 1.5: Garb. Procedures should generally require that personnel wear clean clothing covers that generate low amounts of particles in the controlled area. Clean gowns or closed coats with sleeves that have elastic binding at the cuff are recommended. Hand, finger, and wrist jewelry should be minimized or eliminated. Head and facial hair should be covered. Masks are recommended during aseptic preparation procedures.

Personnel preparing sterile products should scrub their hands and arms (to the elbow) with an appropriate antimicrobial skin cleanser.

RL 1.6: Aseptic technique and product preparation. Sterile products should be prepared with aseptic technique in a Class 100 environment. Personnel should scrub their hands and forearms for an appropriate length of time with a suitable antimicrobial skin cleanser at the beginning of each aseptic compounding process and when re-entering the controlled area. Personnel should wear appropriate attire (see RL 1.5: Garb). Eating, drinking, and smoking should be prohibited in the controlled area. Talking should be minimized in the critical area during aseptic preparation.

Ingredients used to compound sterile products should be determined to be stable, compatible, and appropriate for the product to be prepared, according to manufacturer or USP guidelines or appropriate scientific references. The ingredients of the preparation should be predetermined to be suitable to result in a final product that meets physiological norms for solution osmolality and pH, as appropriate for the intended route of administration. Each ingredient and container should be inspected for defects, expiration date, and product integrity before use. Expired, inappropriately stored, or defective products should not be used in preparing sterile products. Defective products should be promptly reported to the FDA.[30]

Only materials essential for preparing the sterile product should be placed in the laminar-airflow hood. The surfaces of ampuls, vials, and container closures (e.g., vial stoppers) should be disinfected by swabbing or spraying with an appropriate disinfectant solution (e.g., 70% isopropyl alcohol) before placement in the hood. Materials used in aseptic preparation should be arranged in the critical area of the hood in a manner that prevents interruption of the unidirectional airflow between the high-efficiency particulate air (HEPA) filter and critical sites of needles, vials, ampuls, containers, and transfer sets. All aseptic procedures should be performed at least 6 inches inside the front edge of the laminar-airflow hood, in a clear path of unidirectional airflow between the HEPA filter and work materials (e.g., needles, stoppers). The number of personnel preparing sterile products in the hood at one time should be minimized. Overcrowding of the critical work area may interfere with unidirectional airflow and increase the potential for compounding errors. Likewise, the number of units being prepared in the hood at one time should be consistent with the amount of work space in the critical area. Automated compounding devices and other equipment placed in or adjacent to the critical area should be cleaned, disinfected, and placed to avoid contamination or disruption of the unidirectional airflow between the HEPA filter and sterile surfaces.

Aseptic technique should be used to avoid touch contamination of sterile needles, syringe parts (e.g., plunger, syringe tip), and other critical sites. Solutions from ampuls should be properly filtered to remove particles. Solutions of reconstituted powders should be mixed carefully, ensuring complete dissolution of the drug with the appropriate diluent. Needle entry into vials with rubber stoppers should be done cautiously to avoid the creation of rubber core particles. Before, during, and after the preparation of sterile products, the pharmacist should carefully check the identity and verify the amounts of the ingredients in sterile preparations against the original prescription, medication order, or other appropriate documentation (e.g., computerized patient profile, label generated from a pharmacist-verified order) before the product is released or dispensed. Additional information on aseptic technique is available elsewhere.[6,25,31]

For preparation involving automated compounding devices, data entered into the compounding device should be verified by a pharmacist before compounding begins and end-product checks should be performed to verify accuracy of ingredient delivery. These checks may include weighing and visually verifying the final product. For example, the expected weight (in grams) of the final product, based on the specific gravities of the ingredients and their respective volumes, can be documented on the compounding formula sheet, dated, and initialed by the responsible pharmacist. Once compounding is completed, each final product can be weighed and its weight compared with the expected weight. The product's actual weight should fall within a pre-established threshold for variance.[32] Visual verification may be aided by marking the beginning level of each bulk container before starting the automated mixing process and checking each container after completing the mixing process to determine whether the final levels appear reasonable in comparison with expected volumes. The operator should also periodically observe the device during the mixing process to ensure that the device is operating properly (e.g., check to see that all stations are operating).[33] If there are doubts whether a product or component has been properly prepared or stored, then the product should not be used. Refractive index measurements may also be used to verify the addition of certain ingredients.[34]

RL 1.7: Process validation. Validation of aseptic processing procedures provides a mechanism for ensuring that processes consistently result in sterile products of acceptable quality. For most aseptic preparation proce-

dures, process validation is actually a method of assessing the adequacy of a person's aseptic technique. It is recommended that each individual involved in the preparation of sterile products successfully complete a validation process on technique before being allowed to prepare sterile products. The validation process should follow a written procedure that includes evaluation of technique through process simulation.[35-37]

Process simulation testing is valuable for assessing the compounding process, especially aseptic fill operations.[17] It allows for the evaluation of opportunities for microbial contamination during all steps of sterile product preparation. The sterility of the final product is a cumulative function of all processes involved in its preparation and is ultimately determined by the processing step providing the lowest probability of sterility.[38] Process simulation testing is carried out in the same manner as normal production except that an appropriate microbiological growth medium is used in place of the actual products used during sterile preparation. The growth medium is processed as if it were a product being compounded for patient use; the same personnel, procedures, equipment, and materials are involved. The medium samples are then incubated and evaluated. If no microbial growth is detected, this provides evidence that adequate aseptic technique was used. If growth is detected, the entire sterile preparation process must be evaluated, corrective action taken, and the process simulation test performed again.[17,38] No products intended for patient use should be prepared by an individual until the process simulation test indicates that the individual can competently perform aseptic procedures. It is recommended that personnel competency be revalidated at least annually, whenever the quality assurance program yields an unacceptable result, and whenever unacceptable techniques are observed; this revalidation should be documented.

RL 1.8: Expiration dating. All pharmacy-prepared sterile products should bear an appropriate expiration date. The expiration date assigned should be based on currently available drug stability information and sterility considerations. Sources of drug stability information include references (e.g., *Remington's Pharmaceutical Sciences*, *Handbook on Injectable Drugs*), manufacturer recommendations, and reliable, published research. When interpreting published drug stability information, the pharmacist should consider all aspects of the final sterile product being prepared (e.g., drug reservoir, drug concentration, storage conditions).[15,16] Methods used for establishing expiration dates should be documented. Appropriate inhouse (or contract service) stability testing may be used to determine expiration dates.

RL 1.9: Labeling. Sterile products should be labeled with at least the following information:

1 For patient-specific products: the patient's name and any other appropriate patient identification (e.g., location, identification number); for batch-prepared products: control or lot number;
2 All solution and ingredient names, amounts,

strengths, and concentrations (when applicable);
3. Expiration date (and time, when applicable);
4. Prescribed administration regimen, when appropriate (including rate and route of administration);
5. Appropriate auxiliary labeling (including precautions);
6. Storage requirements;
7. Identification (e.g., initials) of the responsible pharmacist;
8. Device-specific instructions (when appropriate); and
9. Any additional information, in accordance with state or federal requirements.

It may also be useful to include a reference number for the prescription or medication order in the labeling; this information is usually required for products dispensed to outpatients. The label should be legible and affixed to the final container in a manner enabling it to be read while the sterile product is being administered (when possible).

RL 1.10: End-product evaluation. The final product should be inspected and evaluated for container leaks, container integrity, solution cloudiness, particulates in the solution, appropriate solution color, and solution volume when preparation is completed and again when the product is dispensed. The responsible pharmacist should verify that the product was compounded accurately with respect to the use of correct ingredients, quantities, containers, and reservoirs; different methods may be used for end-product verification (e.g., observation, calculation checks, documented records).

RL 1.11: Documentation. The following should be documented and maintained on file for an adequate period of time, according to organizational policies and procedures and state regulatory requirements: (1) the training and competency evaluation of employees in sterile product procedures, (2) refrigerator and freezer temperatures, and (3) certification of laminar-airflow hoods. Pharmacists should also maintain appropriate dispensing records for sterile products, in accordance with state regulatory requirements.

Quality assurance for risk level 2

Because the risks associated with contamination of a sterile product are increased with long-term storage and administration, more stringent requirements are appropriate for risk level 2 preparation.

RL 2.1: Policies and procedures. In addition to all recommendations for risk level 1, the written quality assurance program should define and identify necessary environmental monitoring devices and techniques to be used to ensure an adequate environment for risk level 2 sterile product preparation. Examples include the use of airborne particle counters, air velocity and temperature meters, viable particle samplers (e.g., slit samplers), agar plates, and swab sampling of surfaces and potential contamination sites. All aspects of risk level 2 sterile product preparation, storage, and distribution, including details such as the choice of cleaning materials and disinfectants and the monitoring of equipment accuracy, should be addressed in written policies and procedures. Limits of acceptability (threshold or action levels) for environmental monitoring and process simulation and actions to be implemented when thresholds are exceeded should be defined in written policies. For sterile batch compounding, written policies and procedures should be established for the use of master formulas and work sheets and for appropriate documentation. Policies and procedures should also address personnel attire in the controlled area, lot number determination and documentation, and any other quality assurance procedures unique to compounding risk level 2 sterile products.

RL 2.2: Personnel education, training, and evaluation. All recommendations for risk level 1 should be met. In addition to recommendations for risk level 1, assessment of the competency of personnel preparing risk level 2 sterile products should include an appropriate process simulation procedure (as described in RL 1.7: Process validation). However, process simulation procedures for assessing the preparation of risk level 2 sterile products should be representative of all types of manipulations, products, and batch sizes personnel preparing risk level 2 products are likely to encounter.

RL 2.3: Storage and handling. All storage and handling recommendations for risk level 1 should be met.

RL 2.4: Facilities and equipment. In addition to all recommendations for risk level 1, the following are recommended for risk level 2 sterile product preparation:

1. Risk level 2 products should be prepared in a Class 100 horizontal- or vertical-laminar-airflow hood that is properly situated in a controlled area that meets Class 100,000 conditions (or better) for acceptable airborne particle levels. Class 100,000 conditions mean that no more than 100,000 particles 0.5 mm and larger may exist per cubic foot of air.[28] A positive pressure relative to adjacent pharmacy areas is recommended.

2. Cleaning materials (e.g., mops, sponges, germicidal disinfectants) for use in the controlled area or cleanroom should be carefully selected. They should be made of materials that generate a low amount of particles. If reused, cleaning materials should be cleaned and disinfected between uses.

3. The critical-area work surfaces (e.g., interior of the laminar-airflow hood) should be disinfected frequently and before and after each batch preparation process with an appropriate agent, according to written policies and procedures. Floors should be disinfected at least daily. Carpet or porous floors, porous walls, and porous ceiling tiles are not desirable in the controlled area because these surfaces cannot be properly disinfected. Exterior hood surfaces and other hard surfaces in the controlled area, such as shelves, carts, tables, and stools, should be disinfected weekly and after any unanticipated event that could increase the risk of contamination. Walls should be cleaned at least monthly.

4. To ensure that an appropriate environment is maintained for risk level 2 sterile product preparation, an effective written environmental monitoring program is recommended.[26] Sampling of air and surfaces according to a written plan and schedule is recommended.[17,26] The plan

and frequency should be adequate to document that the controlled area is suitable and that the laminar-airflow hood(s) or biological-safety cabinet(s) meet the Class 100 requirements. Limits of acceptability (thresholds or action levels) and appropriate actions to be taken in the event thresholds are exceeded should be specified.

5. To help reduce the number of particles in the controlled area, an adjacent support area (e.g., anteroom) of high cleanliness, separated from the controlled area by a barrier (e.g., plastic curtain, partition, wall), is desirable. Appropriate activities for the support area include, but are not limited to, hand washing, gowning and gloving, removal of packaging and cardboard items, and cleaning and disinfecting hard-surface containers and supplies before placing these items in the controlled area.

RL 2.5: Garb. All recommendations for risk level 1 should be met. Gloves, gowns, and masks are recommended for the preparation of all risk level 2 sterile products. It must be emphasized that, even if sterile gloves are used, gloves do not remain sterile during aseptic compounding; however, they do assist in containing bacteria, skin, and other particles that may be shed, even from scrubbed hands. Clean gowns, coveralls, or closed jackets with sleeves having elastic binding at the cuff are recommended; these garments should be made of low-shedding materials. Shoe covers may be helpful in maintaining the cleanliness of the controlled area. During sterile product preparation, gloves should be rinsed frequently with a suitable agent (e.g., 70% isopropyl alcohol) and changed when their integrity is compromised (i.e., when they are punctured or torn).

RL 2.6: Aseptic technique and product preparation. All recommendations for risk level 1 sterile production preparation should be met.

A master work sheet should be developed for each batch of sterile products to be prepared. Once approved by the designated pharmacist, a verified duplicate (e.g., photocopy) of the master work sheet should be used as the preparation work sheet from which each batch is prepared and on which all documentation for that batch occurs. A separate preparation work sheet should be used for each batch prepared. The master work sheet should consist of the formula, components, compounding directions or procedures, a sample label, and evaluation and testing requirements.[39] The preparation work sheet should be used to document the following:

1. Identity of all solutions and ingredients and their corresponding amounts, concentrations, or volumes;
2. Manufacturer lot number for each component;
3. Component manufacturer or suitable identifying number;
4. Container specifications (e.g., syringe, pump cassette);
5. Lot or control number assigned to batch;
6. Expiration date of batch-prepared products;
7. Date of preparation;
8. Identity (e.g., initials, codes, signatures) of personnel involved in preparation;
9. End-product evaluation and testing specifications;
10. Storage requirements;

11. Specific equipment used during aseptic preparation (e.g., a specific automated compounding device); and
12. Comparison of actual yield to anticipated yield, when appropriate.

A policy and procedure could be developed that allows separate documentation of batch formulas, compounding instructions, and records. However documentation is done, a procedure should exist for easy retrieval of all records pertaining to a particular batch. Each group of sterile batch-prepared products should bear a unique lot number. Under no circumstances should identical lot numbers be assigned to different products or different batches of the same product. Lot numbers may be alphabetic, numeric, or alphanumeric.

The process of combining multiple sterile ingredients into a single, sterile reservoir for subdivision into multiple units for dispensing may necessitate additional quality control procedures. It is recommended that calculations associated with this process be verified by a second pharmacist, when possible; this verification should be documented. Because this process often involves making multiple entries into the intermediate sterile reservoir, the likelihood of contamination may be greater than that associated with the preparation of other risk level 2 sterile products.

RL 2.7: Process validation. Each individual involved in the preparation of risk level 2 sterile products should successfully complete a validation process, as recommended for risk level 1. Process simulation procedures for compounding risk level 2 sterile products should be representative of all types of manipulations, products, and batch sizes that personnel preparing risk level 2 sterile products are likely to encounter.

RL 2.8: Expiration dating. All recommendations for risk level 1 should be met.

RL 2.9: Labeling. All recommendations for risk level 1 should be met.

RL 2.10: End-product evaluation. All recommendations for risk level 1 should be met. Additionally, the growth media fill procedure should be supplemented with a program of end-product sterility testing, according to a formal sampling plan.[40-42] Written policies and procedures should specify measurements and methods of testing. Policies and procedures should include a statistically valid sampling plan and acceptance criteria for the sampling and testing. The criteria should be statistically adequate to reasonably ensure that the entire batch meets all specifications. Products not meeting all specifications should be rejected and discarded. There should be a mechanism for recalling all products of a specific batch if end-product testing procedures yield unacceptable results. On completion of final testing, products should be stored in a manner that ensures their identity, strength, quality, and purity. Detailed information on end-product sterility testing is published elsewhere.[7,16]

RL 2.11: Documentation. All recommendations for risk level 1 should be met. Additionally, documentation of end-product sampling and batch-preparation records should be maintained for an adequate period of time, according to organizational policies and procedures and state regulatory requirements. Documentation for sterile batch-prepared products should include the

1. Master work sheet;
2. Preparation work sheet; and
3. End-product evaluation and testing results.

Quality assurance for risk level 3

General comment on risk level 3. Risk level 3 addresses the preparation of products that pose the greatest potential risk to patients. The quality assurance activities described in this section are clearly more demanding—in terms of processes, facilities, and final product assessment—than for risk levels 1 and 2. Ideally, the activities described for risk level 3 would be used for all high-risk products. The activities may be viewed as most important in circumstances in which the medical need for such high-risk products is *routine.* In circumstances where the medical need for such a product is immediate (and there is not a suitable alternative) or when the preparation of such a product is rare, professional judgment must be applied as to the extent to which some activities (e.g., strict facility design, quarantine and final product testing before product dispensing) should be applied.

RL 3.1: Policies and procedures. There should be written policies and procedures related to every aspect of preparation of risk level 3 sterile products. These policies and procedures should be detailed enough to ensure that all products have the identity, strength, quality, and purity purported for the product.[13,16] All policies and procedures should be reviewed and approved by the designated pharmacist. There should be a mechanism designed to ensure that policies and procedures are communicated, understood, and adhered to by personnel cleaning or working in the controlled area or support area. Policies and procedures should be reviewed at least annually by the designated pharmacist and department head. Written policies and procedures should define and identify the environmental monitoring activities necessary to ensure an adequate environment for risk level 3 sterile product preparation.

In addition to the policies and procedures required for risk levels 1 and 2, there should be written policies and procedures for the following:

1. Component handling and storage;
2. Any additional personnel qualifications commensurate with the preparation of risk level 3 sterile products;
3. Personnel responsibilities in the controlled area (e.g., cleaning, maintenance, access to controlled area);
4. Equipment use, maintenance, calibration, and testing;
5. Sterilization;
6. Master formula and master work sheet development and use;
7. End-product evaluation and testing;
8. Appropriate documentation for preparation of risk level 3 sterile products;
9. Use, control, and monitoring of environmentally con-

trolled areas and calibration of monitoring equipment;
10. Validation of processes for preparing risk level 3 sterile products;
11. Quarantine of products and release from quarantine, if applicable;
12. A mechanism for recall of products from patients in the event that end-product testing procedures yield unacceptable results; and
13. Any other quality control procedures unique to the preparation of risk level 3 sterile products.

RL 3.2: Personnel education, training, and evaluation. Persons preparing sterile products at risk level 3 must have specific education, training, and experience to perform all functions required for the preparation of risk level 3 sterile products. However, final responsibility should lie with the pharmacist, who should be knowledgeable in the principles of good manufacturing practices and proficient in quality assurance requirements, equipment used in the preparation of risk level 3 sterile products, and other aspects of sterile product preparation. The pharmacist should have sufficient education, training, experience, and demonstrated competency to ensure that all sterile products prepared from sterile or nonsterile components have the identity, strength, quality, and purity purported for the products.[7,13] In addition to the body of knowledge required for risk levels 1 and 2, the pharmacist should possess sufficient knowledge in the following areas:

1. Aseptic processing[17,30,43];
2. Quality control and quality assurance as related to environmental, component, and end-product testing;
3. Sterilization techniques[16]; and
4. Container, equipment, and closure system selection.

All pharmacy personnel involved in the cleaning and maintenance of the controlled area should be specially trained and thoroughly knowledgeable in the special requirements of Class 100 critical-area technology and design. There should be documented, ongoing training for all employees to enable retention of expertise.

RL 3.3: Storage and handling. In addition to recommendations for risk levels 1 and 2, risk level 3 policies and procedures for storage and handling should include the procurement, identification, storage, handling, testing, and recall of components and finished products.

Components and finished products ready to undergo end-product testing should be stored in a manner that prevents their use before release by a pharmacist, minimizes the risk of contamination, and enables identification. There should be identifiable storage areas that can be used to quarantine products, if necessary, before they are released.[15]

RL 3.4: Facilities and equipment. Preparation of risk level 3 sterile products should occur in a Class 100 horizontal- or vertical-laminar-airflow hood that is properly situated in a controlled area that meets Class 10,000 conditions for acceptable airborne particle levels *or* in a properly maintained and monitored Class 100 cleanroom (without the hood).[26] The controlled area should have a positive pressure differential relative to adjacent, less clean areas of at least 0.05 inch of water.[17] Solutions that are to be terminally sterilized may be prepared in a Class 100 laminar-airflow hood located inside a controlled area that meets Class 100,000 conditions.

To allow proper cleaning and disinfection, walls, floors, and ceilings in the controlled area should be nonporous. To help reduce the number of particles in the controlled area, an adjacent support area (e.g., anteroom) should be provided.

During the preparation of risk level 3 sterile products, access to the controlled area or cleanroom should be limited to those individuals who are required to be in the area and are properly attired. The environment of the main access areas directly adjacent to the controlled area (e.g., anteroom) should meet at least Federal Standard 209E Class 100,000 requirements.[28] To help maintain a Class 100 critical-area environment during compounding, the adjacent support area (e.g., anteroom) should be separated from the controlled area by a barrier (e.g., plastic curtain, partition, wall). Written policies and procedures for monitoring the environment of the controlled area and adjacent areas should be developed.[17,26]

No sterile products should be prepared in the controlled area if it fails to meet established criteria specified in the policies and procedures. A calibrated particle counter capable of measuring air particles 0.5 µm and larger should be used to monitor airborne particulate matter. Before product preparation begins, the positive-pressure air status should meet or exceed the requirements. Air samples should be taken at several places in the controlled area with the appropriate environmental monitoring devices (e.g., nutrient agar plates). Surfaces on which work actually occurs, including laminar-airflow hood surfaces and tabletops, should be monitored using surface contact plates, the swab–rinse technique, or other appropriate methods.[37,42]

Test results should be reviewed and criteria should be re-established to determine the point at which the preparation of risk level 3 sterile products will be disallowed until corrective measures are taken. When the environment does not meet the criteria specified in the policies and procedures, sterile product processing should immediately cease and corrective action should be taken. In the event that this occurs, written policies and procedures should delineate alternative methods of sterile product preparation to enable timely fulfillment of prescription orders.

Equipment should be adequate to prevent microbiological contamination. Methods should be established for the cleaning, preparation, sterilization, calibration, and documented use of all equipment.

Critical-area work surfaces should be disinfected with an appropriate agent before the preparation of each product. Floors in the controlled area should be disinfected at least daily. Exterior hood surfaces and other hard surfaces in the controlled area, such as shelves, tables, and stools, should be disinfected weekly and after any unanticipated event that could increase the risk of contamination. Walls and ceilings in the controlled area or cleanroom should be

disinfected at least weekly.

Large pieces of equipment, such as tanks, carts, and tables, used in the controlled area or cleanroom should be made of a material that can be easily cleaned and disinfected; stainless steel is recommended. Equipment that does not come in direct contact with the finished product should be properly cleaned, rinsed, and disinfected before being placed in the controlled area. All nonsterile equipment that will come in contact with the sterilized final product should be properly sterilized before introduction into the controlled area; this precaution includes such items as tubing, filters, containers, and other processing equipment. The sterilization process should be monitored and documented.[17]

RL 3.5: Garb. All recommendations for risk levels 1 and 2 should be met. Additionally, cleanroom garb should be worn inside the controlled area at all times during the preparation of risk level 3 sterile products. Attire should consist of a low-shedding coverall, head cover, face mask, and shoe covers. These garments may be either disposable or reusable. Head and facial hair should be covered. Before donning these garments over street clothes, personnel should thoroughly wash their hands and arms up to the elbows with a suitable antimicrobial skin cleanser.[19] Sterile disposable gloves should be worn and rinsed frequently with an appropriate agent (e.g., 70% isopropyl alcohol) during processing. The gloves should be changed if the integrity is compromised. If persons leave the controlled area *or support area* during processing, they should regown with clean garments before re-entering.

RL 3.6: Aseptic technique and product preparation. All recommendations for risk levels 1 and 2 should be met. Methods should ensure that components and containers remain free from contamination and are easily identified as to the product, lot number, and expiration date. If components are not finished sterile pharmaceuticals obtained from licensed manufacturers, pharmacists should ensure that these components meet USP standards. Products prepared from nonsterile ingredients should be tested to ensure that they do not exceed specified endotoxin limits.[16] As each new lot of components and containers is received, the components should be quarantined until properly identified, tested, or verified by a pharmacist.

The methods for preparing sterile products and using process controls should be designed to ensure that finished products have the identity, strength, quality, and purity they are intended to have. Any deviations from established methods should be documented and appropriately justified.

A master work sheet should be developed for the preparation of each risk level 3 sterile product. Once approved by the pharmacist, a verified duplicate of the master work sheet should be used as the controlling document from which each sterile end product or batch of prepared products is compounded and on which all documentation for that product or batch occurs. The master work sheet should document all the requirements for risk level 2 plus the following:

1. Comparison of actual with anticipated yield;
2. Sterilization method(s); and
3. Quarantine specifications.

The preparation work sheet should serve as the batch record for each time a risk level 3 sterile product is prepared. Each batch of pharmacy-prepared sterile products should bear a unique lot number, as described in risk level 2.

There should be documentation on the preparation work sheet of all additions of individual components plus the signatures or initials of those individuals involved with the measuring or weighing and addition of these components.

The selection of the final packaging system (including container and closure) for the sterile product is crucial to maintaining product integrity. To the extent possible, presterilized containers obtained from licensed manufacturers should be used. If an aseptic filling operation is used, the container should be sterile at the time of the filling operation. If nonsterile containers are used, methods for sterilizing these containers should be established. Final containers selected should be capable of maintaining product integrity (i.e., identity, strength, quality, and purity) throughout the shelf life of the product.[44]

For products requiring sterilization, selection of an appropriate method of sterilization is of prime importance. Methods of product sterilization include sterile filtration, autoclaving, dry heat sterilization, chemical sterilization, and irradiation.[16,45] Selection of the sterilization technique should be based on the properties of the product being processed. The pharmacist must ensure that the sterilization method used is appropriate for the product components and does not alter the pharmaceutical properties of the final product. A method of sterilization often used by pharmacists is sterile filtration.[46] In sterile filtration, the product should be filtered into presterilized containers under aseptic conditions. Sterilizing filters of 0.22 µm or smaller porosity should be used in this process. Colloidal or viscous products may require use of a 0.45-µm filter; however, extreme caution should be exercised in these circumstances, and more stringent end-product sterility testing is essential.[26,47,48]

To ensure that a bacteria-retentive filter did not rupture during filtration of a product, an integrity test should be performed on all filters immediately after filtration. This test may be accomplished by performing a bubble point test, in which pressurized gas is applied to the upstream side of the filter with the downstream outlet immersed in water and the pressure at which a steady stream of bubbles begins to appear is noted.[46,48] The observed pressure is then compared with the manufacturer's specification for the filter. To compare the used filter with the manufacturer's specifications, which would be based on the filtration of water through the filter, it is necessary to first rinse the filter with sterile water for injection. An observed value lower than the manufacturer's specification indicates that the filter was defective or ruptured during the sterilization process. Methods should be established for handling, testing, and resterilizing any product processed with a filter that fails the integrity test.

RL 3.7: Process validation. In addition to risk level 1 and 2 recommendations, written policies and procedures should be established to validate all processes involved in the preparation of risk level 3 sterile products (including all procedures, equipment, and techniques) from sterile or nonsterile components. In addition to evaluating personnel technique, process validation provides a mechanism for determining whether a particular process will, when performed by qualified personnel, consistently produce the intended results.

RL 3.8: Expiration dating. In addition to risk level 2 recommendations, there should be reliable methods for establishing all expiration dates including laboratory testing of products for sterility, pyrogenicity, and chemical content, when necessary. These tests should be conducted in a manner based on appropriate statistical criteria, and the results documented.

RL 3.9: Labeling. All recommendations for risk levels 1 and 2 should be met.

RL 3.10: End-product evaluation. For each preparation of a sterile product or a batch of sterile products, there should be appropriate laboratory determination of conformity with established written specifications and policies. Any reprocessed material should undergo complete final product testing. It is advisable to quarantine sterile products compounded from nonsterile components, pending the results of end-product testing. If products prepared from nonsterile components must be dispensed before satisfactory completion of end-product testing, there must be a procedure to allow for immediate recall of the products from patients to whom they were dispensed.

RL 3.11: Documentation. In addition to the recommendations for risk levels 1 and 2, documentation for risk level 3 sterile products should include

1. Preparation work sheet;
2. Sterilization records of final products (if applicable);
3. Quarantine records (if applicable); and
4. End-product evaluation and testing results.

___

[a]Unless otherwise stated in this document, the term "sterile products" refers to sterile drug or nutritional substances that are prepared (e.g., compounded or repackaged) by pharmacy personnel.

Appendix A—Glossary

Aseptic preparation: The technique involving procedures designed to preclude contamination (of drugs, packaging, equipment, or supplies) by microorganisms during processing.

Batch preparation: Compounding of multiple sterile-product units, in a single discrete process, by the, same individual(s), carried out during one limited time period.

Cleanroom: A room in which the concentration of airborne particles is controlled and there are one or more clean zones.

(A clean zone is a defined space in which the concentration of airborne particles is controlled to meet a specified airborne-particulate cleanliness class.) Cleanrooms are classified based on the maximum number of allowable particles 0.5 μm and larger per cubic foot of air. For example, the air particle count in a Class 100 cleanroom may not exceed a total of 100 particles of 0.5 μm and larger per cubic foot of air.[28]

Closed-system transfer: The movement of sterile products from one container to another in which the container-closure system and transfer devices remain intact throughout the entire transfer process, compromised only by the penetration of a sterile, pyrogen-free needle or cannula through a designated stopper or port to effect transfer, withdrawal, or delivery. Withdrawal of a sterile solution from an ampul in a Class 100 environment would generally be considered acceptable; however, the use of a rubber-stoppered vial, when available, would be preferable.

Compounding: For purposes of this document, compounding simply means the mixing of substances to prepare a medication for patient use. This activity would include dilution, admixture, repackaging, reconstitution, and other manipulations of sterile products.

Controlled area: For purposes of this document, a controlled area is the area designated for preparing sterile products.

Critical areas: Any area in the controlled area where products or containers are exposed to the environment.[37]

Critical site: An opening providing a direct pathway between a sterile product and the environment or any surface coming in contact with the product or environment.

Critical surface: Any surface that comes into contact with previously sterilized products or containers.[37]

Expiration date: The date (and time, when applicable) beyond which a product should not be used (i.e., the product should be discarded beyond this date and time). NOTE: Circumstances may occur in which the expiration date and time arrive while an infusion is in progress. When this occurs, judgment should be applied in determining whether it is appropriate to discontinue that infusion and replace the product. Organizational policies on this should be clear.

HEPA filter: A high-efficiency particulate air (HEPA) filter composed of pleats of filter medium separated by rigid sheets of corrugated paper or aluminum foil that direct the flow of air forced through the filter in a uniform parallel flow. HEPA filters remove 99.97% of all air particles 0.3 μm or larger. When HEPA filters are used as a component of a horizontal- or vertical-laminar-airflow hood, an environment can be created consistent with standards for a Class 100 cleanroom.[40]

Quality assurance: For purposes of this document, quality assurance is the set of activities used to ensure that the processes used in the preparation of sterile drug products lead to products that meet predetermined standards of quality.

Quality control: For purposes of this document, quality control is the set of testing activities used to determine that the ingredients, components (e.g., containers), and final sterile products prepared meet predetermined requirements with respect to identity, purity, nonpyrogenicity, and sterility.

Repackaging: The subdivision or transfer from a container or device to a different container or device, such as a syringe or ophthalmic container.

Sterilizing filter: A filter that, when challenged with a solution containing the microorganism *Pseudomonas diminuta*, at a minimum concentration of 10^7 organisms per square centimeter of filter surface, will produce a sterile effluent.[16,17]

Temperatures (USP): Frozen means temperatures between −20 and −10 °C (−4 and 14 °F). Refrigerated means temperatures between 2 and 8 °C (36 and 46 °F). Room temperature means temperatures between 15 and 30 °C (59 and 86 °F).[16]

Validation: Documented evidence providing a high degree of assurance that a specific process will consistently produce a product meeting its predetermined specifications and quality attributes.[17]

References

1. Hughes CF, Grant AF, Leckie BD et al. Cardioplegic solution: a contamination crisis. *J Thorac Cardiovasc Surg.* 1986; 91:296-302.
2. Associated Press. Pittsburgh woman loses eye to tainted drugs; 12 hurt. *Baltimore Sun.* 1990; Nov 9:3A.
3. Anon. ASHP gears up multistep action plan regarding sterile drug products. *Am J Hosp Pharm.* 1991; 48:386,389-90. News.
4. Dugleaux G, Coutour XL, Hecquard C et al. Septicemia caused by contaminated parenteral nutrition pouches: the refrigerator as an unusual cause. *J Parenter Enter Nutr.* 1991; 15:474-5.
5. Solomon SL, Khabbaz RF, Parker RH et al. An outbreak of *Candida parapsilosis* bloodstream infections in patients receiving parenteral nutrition. *J Infect Dis.* 1984; 149:98-102.
6. National Coordinating Committee on Large Volume Parenterals. Recommended methods for compounding intravenous admixtures in hospitals. *Am J Hosp Pharm.* 1975; 32:261-70.
7. National Coordinating Committee on Large Volume Parenterals. Recommended guidelines for quality assurance in hospital centralized intravenous admixture services. *Am J Hosp Pharm.* 1980; 37:645-55.
8. National Coordinating Committee on Large Volume Parenterals. Recommendations for the labeling of large volume parenterals. *Am J Hosp Pharm.* 1978; 35:49-51.
9. National Coordinating Committee on Large Volume Parenterals. Recommended standard of practice, policies, and procedures for intravenous therapy. *Am J Hosp Pharm.* 1980; 37:660-3.
10. National Coordinating Committee on Large Volume Parenterals. Recommended procedures for in-use testing of large volume parenterals suspected of contamination or of producing a reaction in a patient. *Am J Hosp Pharm.* 1978; 35:678-82.
11. National Coordinating Committee on Large Volume Parenterals. Recommended system for surveillance and reporting of problems with large volume parenterals in hospitals. *Am J Hosp Pharm.* 1975; 34:1251-3.
12. Barker KN, ed. Recommendations of the NCCLVP for the compounding and administration of intravenous solutions. Bethesda, MD: American Society of Hospital Pharmacists; 1981.
13. Joint Commission on Accreditation of Healthcare Organizations. 1993 Accreditation manual for hospitals. Oakbrook Terrace, IL: Joint Commission on Accreditation of Healthcare Organizations; 1992.
14. Joint Commission on Accreditation of Healthcare Organizations. 1993 Accreditation manual for home care. Vol. 1. Standards. Oakbrook Terrace, IL: Joint Commission on Accreditation of Healthcare Organizations; 1993.
15. Food and Drug Administration. Title 21 Code of Federal Regulations. Part 21—current good manufacturing practice for finished pharmaceuticals. United States.
16. The United States pharmacopeia, 22nd rev., and The national formulary, 17th ed. Rockville, MD: The United States Pharmacopeial Convention; 1989.
17. Division of Manufacturing and Product Quality, Office of Compliance, Food and Drug Administration. Guideline on sterile drug products produced by aseptic processing. Rockville, MD:

Food and Drug Administration; 1987.

18. Centers for Disease Control. Guideline for prevention of intravascular infections. *Am J Infect Control.* 1983; 11(5):183-93.

19. Centers for Disease Control. Guideline for handwashing and hospital environmental control. *Am J Infect Control.* 1986; 4(8):110-29.

20. Anon. Sterile drug products for home use. *Pharmacopeial Forum.* 1993; 19:5380-409.

21. Stiles ML, Tu Y-H, Allen LV Jr. Stability of morphine sulfate in portable pump reservoirs during storage and simulated administration. *Am J Hosp Pharm.* 1989; 46:1404-7.

22. Duafala ME, Kleinberg ML, Nacov C et al. Stability of morphine sulfate in infusion devices and containers for intravenous administration. *Am J Hosp Pharm.* 1990; 47:143-6.

23. Seidel AM. Quality control for parenteral nutrition compounding. Paper presented at 48th ASHP Annual Meeting; San Diego, CA: 1991 Jun 6.

24. American Society of Hospital Pharmacists. ASHP technical assistance bulletin on handling cytotoxic and hazardous drugs. *Am J Hosp Pharm.* 1990; 47:1033-49.

25. American Society of Hospital Pharmacists. Aseptic preparation of parenteral products. (Videotape and study guide.) Bethesda, MD: American Society of Hospital Pharmacists; 1985.

26. Avis KE, Lachman L, Lieberman HA, eds. Pharmaceutical dosage forms: parenteral medications. Vol 2. New York: Marcel Dekker; 1992.

27. American Society of Hospital Pharmacists. ASHP technical assistance bulletin on outcome competencies and training guidelines for institutional pharmacy technician training programs. *Am J Hosp Pharm.* 1982; 39:317-20.

28. Federal Standard No. 209E. Airborne particulate cleanliness classes in cleanrooms and clean zones. Washington, DC: General Services Administration; 1992.

29. Bryan D, Marback RC. Laminar-airflow equipment certification: what the pharmacist needs to know. *Am J Hosp Pharm.* 1984; 41:1343-9.

30. Kessler DA. MedWatch: the new FDA medical products reporting program. *Am J Hosp Pharm.* 1993; 50:1921-36.

31. Hunt ML. Training manual for intravenous admixture personnel, 4th ed. Chicago: Baxter Healthcare Corporation and Pluribus Press, Inc.; 1989.

32. Murphy C. Ensuring accuracy in the use of automatic compounders. *Am J Hosp Pharm.* 1993; 50:60. Letter.

33. Brushwood DB. Hospital liable for defect in cardioplegia solution. *Am J Hosp Pharm.* 1992; 49:1174-6.

34. Meyer GE, Novielli KA, Smith JE. Use of refractive index measurement for quality assurance of pediatric parenteral nutrition solutions. *Am J Hosp Pharm.* 1987; 44:1617-20.

35. Morris BG, Avis KN, Bowles GC. Quality-control plan for intravenous admixture programs. II: validation of operator technique. *Am J Hosp Pharm.* 1980; 37:668-72.

36. Dirks I, Smith FM, Furtado D et al. Method for testing aseptic technique of intravenous admixture personnel. *Am J Hosp Pharm.* 1982; 39:457-9.

37. Brier KL. Evaluating aseptic technique of pharmacy personnel. *Am J Hosp Pharm.* 1983; 40:400-3.

38. Validation of aseptic filling for solution drug products. Technical monograph no. 2. Philadelphia: Parenteral Drug Association, Inc.; 1980.

39. Boylan JC. Essential elements of quality control. *Am J Hosp Pharm.* 1983; 40:1936-9.

40. Choy FN, Lamy PP, Burkhart VD et al. Sterility-testing program for antibiotics and other intravenous admixtures. *Am J Hosp Pharm.* 1982; 39:452-6.

41. Doss HL, James JD, Killough DM et al. Microbiologic quality assurance for intravenous admixtures in a small hospital. *Am J Hosp Pharm.* 1982; 39:832-5.

42. Posey LM, Nutt RE, Thompson PD. Comparison of two methods for detecting microbial contamination in intravenous fluids. *Am J Hosp Pharm.* 1982; 28:659-62.

43. Frieben WR. Control of aseptic processing environment. *Am J Hosp Pharm.* 1983; 40:1928-35.

44. Neidich RL. Selection of containers and closure systems for injectable products. *Am J Hosp Pharm.* 1983; 40:1924-7.

45. Phillips GB, O'Neill M. Sterilization. In: Gennaro AR, ed. Remington's pharmaceutical sciences. 18th ed. Easton, PA: Mack Publishing; 1990:1470-80.

46. McKinnon BT, Avis KE. Membrane filtration of pharmaceutical solutions. *Am J Hosp Pharm.* 1993; 50:1921-36.

47. Olson W. Sterilization of small-volume parenteral and therapeutic proteins by filtration. In: Olson W, Groves MJ, eds. Aseptic pharmaceutical manufacturing: technology for the 1990s. Prairie View, IL: Interpharm; 1987:101-49.

48. Eudailey WA. Membrane filters and membrane filtration processes for health care. *Am J Hosp Pharm.* 1983; 40:1921-3.

49. Turco S, King RE. Extemporaneous preparation. In: Turco S, King RE, eds. Sterile dosage forms. Philadelphia: Lea & Febiger; 1987:55-61.